MW00973318

A Time To HEAR

A Time To HELP

A Time To HEAR

A Time To HELP

LISTENING TO PEOPLE WITH CANCER

DANIEL ROSENBLUM, M.D.

Foreword by Bernard S. Siegel, M.D.

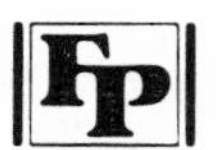

THE FREE PRESS
A Division of Macmillan, Inc.
NEW YORK

Maxwell Macmillan Canada
TORONTO

Maxwell Macmillan International
NEW YORK OXFORD SINGAPORE SYDNEY

The Free Press
A Division of Macmillan, Inc.
866 Third Avenue, New York, N. Y. 10022

Maxwell Macmillan Canada, Inc.
1200 Eglinton Avenue East
Suite 200
Don Mills, Ontario M3C 3N1

Macmillan, Inc. is part of the Maxwell Communication Group of Companies.

Printed in the United States of America

printing number
1 2 3 4 5 6 7 8 9 10

Library of Congress Cataloging-in-Publication Data
Rosenblum, Daniel.
A time to hear, a time to help: listening to people with cancer /
Daniel Rosenblum.
p. cm.
ISBN 0-02-927105-3
1. Cancer—Psychological aspects. 2. Caring. I. Title.
RC262.R66 1993
616.99'4'0019—dc20 92-38162
CIP

The author acknowledges permission to use the following material:

Poem #288, in *The Complete Poems of Emily Dickinson,* edited by Thomas H. Johnson. Copyright © 1929 by Martha Dickinson Bianchi; copyright renewed 1957 by Mary L. Hampson. By permission of Little, Brown and Company.

"Out, Out . . ." and "The Road Not Taken," in *The Poetry of Robert Frost,* edited by Edward Connery Lathem. Copyright © 1969 by Holt, Rinehart and Winston. Reprinted by permission of Henry Holt and Company, Inc.

A Time to Hear, A Time to Help is based on my experiences as a practicing oncologist. My patients have given me consent to use the clinical information presented here because they join me in wishing to help others cope with one of life's greatest challenges. Nevertheless, to protect their privacy, I have changed names, transposed events, merged the stories of different people, and altered identifying characteristics.

To the memory of my father
HASKELL BENJAMIN ROSENBLUM, M.D.
who gave his life for our country in September 1942
and to my mother
JANETH RAVNER ROSENBLUM
who has made giving of herself a way of life.

CONTENTS

FOREWORD

Dr. Daniel Rosenblum's *A Time to Hear, a Time to Help* is an enormous resource for everyone—physicians, patients, and their families—who must deal with cancer. But in addition, it is as great a help to people trying to cope with adversity or afflictions of any kind.

Dr. Rosenblum shows us the true meaning of the word doctor: it is to be a teacher. And we, as patients or sufferers, can learn from him that the dreadful error of seeing disease as punishment can be changed through the process of listening and healing.

Anatole Broyard, who died of cancer and shared his deepest understanding in his book *Intoxicated by My Illness*, wrote that "every patient needs mouth-to-mouth resuscitation, for talk is the kiss of life." Yet if no one is listening, of what value is the talk? If we are deaf to each other's words, we isolate ourselves. Dr. Rosenblum teaches us how to hear each other.

Having, for a time, lived the disease of being a doctor who was trained to treat afflictions, but not people, I know that both the physician and the patient need healing. I like to think of the relationship of patient and doctor as akin to that of "war buddies"—

in the thick of conflict, struggle, and difficulty, but always buddies carrying on the fight together.

Cancer, as experience and as metaphor, is explored in the story of each patient we visit with Dr. Rosenblum. And we see how, in some ways, cancer gives us permission to finally live our unique life.

Helping healing to occur through sharing, dialogue, and a willingness to hear what the other is saying is something most doctors, health workers, and families are not trained to do.

I therefore urge both the physician and the layman to reflect on their own and others' experience as Dr. Rosenblum has done, and to learn this most simple and yet most difficult skill, how to listen. The result will be a new freedom from failure and guilt, and a realization that loving laughter, like hope, can be a welcome bond and healer for us all. When patients, physicians, nurses, and loving friends all become each others' doctor, or teacher, all are better off—for life without words, as Helen Keller said, "is darker by far than blindness."

If you are a patient, caregiver, or doctor, this book will guide you on your path to hearing, helping, and ultimately healing your life—even in the presence of the incurable. Cancer can be beaten by the right "war buddies" affirming friendships, care, and love even at life's darkest moments.

BERNARD S. SIEGEL, M.D.

A Time To HEAR

A Time To HELP

INTRODUCTION

I AM just old enough to remember the 1940s, when children were still punished for saying "bad words." After a mouthful of soap, expletives left a bitter impression not easily forgotten.

In those days, "cancer" was a bad word, too. People avoided saying "cancer" as if it were unmentionable, as if uttering the very name of the disease enabled it to spread. As an adult, I thought the days when cancer was considered bad had vanished. I believed we had entered a new era when the President's cancerous colon was publicly discussed.

I was wrong.

People still shun cancer. When friends get cancer, we wall them off or treat them as if they had "special" needs. We drop our voices, ostracize them, or, worse yet, become overly solicitous. Too easily we forget our membership in the same human family. When one of us has cancer, to some degree it affects all of us, whether we acknowledge its reality or play a game of mental peekaboo. As one of many who have devoted their lives to confronting cancer, I believe more of us should overcome our superstitions and respond to the human needs which surround us.

Cancer is a remarkably egalitarian disease. It has afflicted humanity since prehistoric times. Its character has changed with social movements, dietary patterns, occupational exposures, habits, and environmental conditions, but there is a remarkably constant age-related incidence of cancer throughout the world. At present, because of our relative healthiness, because we survive many of the illnesses which kill younger humans elsewhere, cancer will appear in one out of three of us, and one out of six of us will die from it.

We are not totally insensitive to cancer's presence in our midst. When the American Cancer Society asks for a donation, we readily give. Then we forget about cancer until the telephone rings. The caller tells us our good friend BeeJay is in the hospital. A biopsy. Bad news. Of a sudden, cancer has come home.

"BeeJay! Oh, my God! Not BeeJay!"

We send a card. Or call. After BeeJay's anesthesia wears off, we pay a visit. We're full of sympathy, of course.

Our conversation is strained. We do not know whether to ask for facts about her cancer or to listen to her complaints: The hospital food is inedible! The cleaning service doesn't! The room costs a fortune and the telephone doesn't even work!

So we sit for a while, upset by the anger in BeeJay's voice. It almost seems as if she is angry at *us*!

Later, there's a hint of tears. Not about the cancer (we could understand *that*!), but about BeeJay's cat, SuSu, who is twelve years old and on his last legs and has no one to care for him when the cancer takes its expected toll. "Forget the cat!" we think. But BeeJay can't forget the cat. Indeed, it seems as if SuSu is more important to BeeJay than we are. It almost seems as if BeeJay found less comfort from our visit than from thinking about a dumb animal named SuSu, whom we never really liked, if truth be told, because cat hairs brought on allergies we had tried in vain to hide. Embarrassed at our foolishness, we cut the visit short. Later, while at table with the healthy (thank God!) significant other in our lives, we recount the story of our visit, taking pains to emphasize the discomfort we felt when BeeJay was angry, how we felt like crying when BeeJay cried but kept up a cheerful face, and how completely distracted BeeJay seemed from thinking about the cancer and what could be done about it.

"You'd think BeeJay would be using more energy to work on the cancer!" we say. "No wonder the doctors are worried! What an attitude! I'm disappointed."

So we buy a book. Not for ourselves, but for BeeJay. The body is ailing, the mind must need improving. "Recuperating in the hospital, an excellent time to read," we think. We drop by with the book. There are nurses in the room. BeeJay just came back from X-ray and needs help getting out of the wheelchair. There's been an accident of sorts. The intravenous went dry. BeeJay's arm is sore. It's black and blue from needle sticks. We plan to stay, but it's late. Besides, we only wanted to drop off the book. We didn't know what to say.

The weeks go by. We call from time to time. BeeJay has lots of complaints, sounds almost irritable at times. At others, we're struck by her "marvelous attitude," her willingness to confront the challenge, her courage. But we don't know what to say in return, so the gaps between our calls increase.

Months pass. BeeJay grows worse. We hear about it from a mutual friend. Guilt-stricken, we call again but are afraid to hear the details. It's not the same as the time when BeeJay's water pipes burst during a winter freeze some years ago.

Then we were glad to let BeeJay camp out in our living room. We had lots of time to talk. We adored BeeJay's elegant stir-fry dinners. We let SuSu live in our basement. We had a sense of camaraderie which made us welcome the chance to share the adversity. Now it's our duty to call. BeeJay seems to regard it as her duty to respond. But we avoid talking about the things that matter most to us.

What is it about friendship that makes words flow easiest when they are least essential and ties our tongues at life's most critical moments? What is it about love that makes us prefer honesty and directness about inconsequential matters yet bids us avoid the issues of greatest magnitude? What is it about our hearts that enables us to show them openly on sunny days but leads us, Hamlet-like, into ponderous internal debates when storm clouds loom overhead?

Caught in a web of ambivalence, we feel a need to talk to BeeJay, but words fail us as we weigh the consequences of lending substance to our thoughts through utterance. Death is looming large. BeeJay's parents still don't know. How will the cancer affect the divorce? What about the island summer home we've shared for years? What are we to do?

A Time to Hear, A Time to Help portrays people with cancer and the issues cancer raised in their lives. It describes human reactions to severe illness. Despite similarities in our reactions, we each have unique personalities and points of view; each has a history, a set of friends and relatives, a social role, an identifiable position in the human family. When cancer appears, we are powered by shared feelings and responses: anger, anxiety, denial, a need for information and self-esteem, a will to fight, and the knowledge that a time will come when we can fight no more.

The person with cancer is not the only needy individual. When we visited BeeJay, we had needs, too. We were frightened by an illness, angry because our friend would die. BeeJay's cancer threatened *us* because we were forced to admit that we, too, could get cancer. We wanted to understand, to help, to *do* something about BeeJay's problems. But no one trained us for the role of listener. No one told us how to hear.

We learn to hear by making ourselves available, by listening and caring. People with illness are effective teachers. From somewhere inside the tangle of the disjointed thoughts that constitute awareness of the body's malfunction come groans and screams and finally words that tell us how it feels. The language is foreign at first, but by sticking with it, we learn to understand. In silence, often, we learn, because hearing requires time, attention, commitment, and a willingness to accept whatever comes.

When BeeJay was worried about SuSu, why *not* listen to her complaint? Perhaps we could help SuSu find a home. Perhaps we could hear about the love BeeJay felt for SuSu. Perhaps BeeJay's lament for SuSu was a metaphor for BeeJay's own life. Who knows? *We* certainly won't if we don't give time to it.

An old riddle still amuses a physicist I know. "If a tree falls in the wilderness and there's no one to hear it, does it make a noise?" I'll answer it with yet another. "How can I get relief when I'm angry if no one listens to me yelling?"

When BeeJay exploded because the telephone did not work, we could tell the anger was "inappropriate." We knew BeeJay had handled minor problems calmly in the past. But it was not the past, and the anger was deep and pervasive, coloring even the most ordinary irritations of the daily scene. We heard the anger, but we could not bring ourselves to add, "What are you going to do about it?" and wait for an answer.

We gave BeeJay a book when she got cancer so she could "work on her attitude." We thought she could benefit from the author's suggestions for self-improvement. We were wrong. BeeJay didn't have time to read because every few minutes someone came into her room with a probe, a pen, or a pill. Besides, she was exhausted from lack of sleep and recuperating from surgery.

But how about us? Could our minds stand the "in-depth" exposure BeeJay is getting every day? Could we tolerate the intensity of the experience? We were BeeJay's friends. If we expected courage from BeeJay, we should have demanded no less from ourselves.

Come with me as I go upon my rounds. Meet my friends. They were starngers to me, too, a short while ago, but their cancers brought me into contact with them and their families.

The stories will be difficult to read at first. But we'll be gentle on your feelings, we'll respect your tenderness. We only ask you to respect our feelings in return. Some of us will die before the book is finished, others will be restored to health. But all of us wanted to share our stories with you.

> Don't spurn us, cast us off, or try to shirk
> Our call to help. You've less than we to fear.
> Don't hide from us or scurry back to "work,"
> But listen with your heart a while and hear!

1
BEGINNINGS

> To every thing there is a season,
> and a time to every purpose under heaven: . . .
> A time to keep silence, and a time to speak.
> —Ecclesiastes 3

"WHAT are you going to tell my husband?" Ginny asked me. Her tears had dried, but her voice rose as she spoke. "More important, *how* are you going to tell him? You may know a lot about cancer, but I know a lot about Toby. This is not going to be easy."

Not easy! That was an understatement. The two of us had spent the previous hour talking about Toby's lung cancer. We had been corralled in a conference room with two nurses. Across the hall, in a glassed-in compartment, Toby slept. It had been his first few hours of sleep since his admission to the intensive care unit. Although I had very much wanted him to be part of our conference, I had not had the heart to wake him. Besides, it had been my first opportunity to speak with his wife. Though we had finished our discussion, we could no longer avoid telling Toby the painful facts.

"I've never seen him look so frightened," Ginny said. "He's usually the strong one."

Toby's anxiety had been obvious ever since he heard the words "you have lung cancer." His body shook. His voice trembled. He seemed on the verge of tears. He jumped at every comment, dissected each tiny tidbit of information. But while his mind appeared to be at a heightened state of alertness, he scrambled information instead of clarifying it.

Ginny told me what had happened when the lung specialist, Dr. Starch, came to visit Toby on the previous Friday.

"You have lung cancer, Mr. Thompson," Dr. Starch said.

He spoke as if he expected Toby to understand. Toby was an engineer, an expert in his field. Despite the miscommunication of the past few months, Dr. Starch was certain Toby knew enough about cancer to grasp the implications quickly.

"But I haven't been sick. This is all so sudden."

"Maybe you didn't realize you were sick. I think you had symptoms of cancer several months ago."

"But what about all the tests you did last summer? You told me there were no signs of cancer."

"The tests were wrong. The cancer was too small to see."

"Can it be cured?"

"I doubt it."

"Then what's going to happen to me?"

Dr. Starch turned his eyes.

"Am I . . . am I . . . am I going to die?"

"Probably."

"How soon?"

"Six months, maybe . . ."

Toby looked panicked. He sat erect in his bed in the cardiac intensive care unit. He was drenched with sweat. He looked as if he wanted to cry but couldn't. The racing of his heartbeat was reflected in the dancing squiggle of light on the cardiac monitor above his head. Dr. Starch glanced at his watch.

"I'm sorry. I've got to leave. I'm on a tight schedule this morning. I'm late already. I'll ask Dr. Rosenblum to tell you more about your cancer."

"Who is he?"

"An oncologist . . . a cancer doctor."

9

BEGINNINGS

"Why him?"

"You have lung cancer, Mr. Thompson. It's his specialty."

"Really? It sounds like an awful specialty."

Immediately after talking to Toby, Dr. Starch paged me in the hospital. Fifteen minutes later, we stood together in the hall outside Toby's room.

"I feel a little embarrassed about this diagnosis, Dan," Dr. Starch told me. "I first saw Toby Thompson six months ago. He's a sixty-one-year-old executive in a computer firm. In fact, he's been traveling through eastern Europe in the past several months teaching computer programmers about capitalism. He's highly regarded for his ability to think clearly and to express himself well. He's also a jogger. Six months ago he came to me with an annoying cough. I guess he'd had it about three or four weeks by then. By the time he arrived in my office he was coughing every fifteen minutes. Occasionally, bright red blood would appear. As you know, the usual explanation for this symptom is bronchitis. I thought about cancer, of course, but I did my best to rule it out. He wasn't a smoker, at least he hadn't been for twenty-seven years. I took a chest X ray and a CAT scan of his chest. I saw some old scar tissue in his left lung. He had a severe case of pneumonia as a child. We saw nothing new. Just to make certain, I even did a bronchoscopy. Nothing showed."

"Even by bronchoscopy?"

"I examined every part of his bronchial tree. One branch on the left side showed some inflammation. I think the blood was coming from there. I took specimens but none contained any cancer cells. I thought he had bronchitis. I gave him cough medicine and antibiotics and told him to call me if his symptoms got worse. I did not hear from him again until last week when a cardiologist called me."

I could see the anguish in Dr. Starch's face. I know him to be a careful doctor. He had done everything right. Even so, it had not worked out.

"I still can't quite understand why he never called me. He was getting worse and worse, and yet he continued to act as if my diagnosis of bronchitis explained everything. How could he have done that?"

I shrugged.

"Perhaps it is not hard to understand. Toby's a jogger. He ran in the Marine Corps Marathon when he was in his fifties. He finished in the top half. As long as he could keep on running, he probably believed he wasn't seriously ill. He noticed he lacked stamina. He had been able to run six miles a year ago. Two weeks before he came into the hospital, he could only walk two miles. He knew something was wrong, so he went back to his internist who sent him to a cardiologist. I suppose he thought it was heart failure, but the cardiologist recognized immediately that he had something very different wrong with him. He had fluid around his heart and in his left chest cavity. The "scar" tissue in the left upper lung had gotten bigger. I was certain it was cancer.

"We took specimens from both sources yesterday. This morning the pathologist told me he has cancer."

As we spoke, Dr. Starch stood with his back to the open door of Toby's room. It was my first glimpse of my prospective patient. Through the door I could see him sitting bolt upright in bed. Tubing twisted around his body like the snakes on a caduceus. At a distance of twenty feet, I could tell he was trembling.

"I just told him what we found," Dr. Starch said. "Now it's up to you."

So it was to be my task to talk to Toby. I would have to find a way to help him live with as much strength and dignity as possible for whatever time remained for him. I would have to find a way to ease the emotional burden. I would have to find a way to meet his every expectation. I would have to do all of these things for Toby, and I didn't even know him.

I entered his room with a sense of foreboding. I felt the intensity of his anxiety, which seemed to electrify the air. I wanted to sit beside his bed to ease the tension, but there was no chair. Although the sparse furnishings suited the style of the intensive care unit, they frustrated my need to place us both at ease.

At close range, I could see Toby had undergone several procedures. He had tubes in his chest, his arm, his nose, his bladder. Urine and blood-tinged fluid drained towards the end of his bed while oxygen flowed into his nose from a wall fixture. Thin electric wires were connected from his chest to a monitor.

"What the hell is happening to me?" he asked. His tongue stuck to the roof of his mouth. "I have always been proud of my health. I'm a competitive runner. I knew I had slowed down. I thought it might be my heart. I've had trouble with my blood pressure. I've been taking medicine for years. I thought maybe the doctor should change the medicine. Maybe then my energy would come back. But the cardiologist took one look at me and sent for Dr. Starch. This morning, Dr. Starch told me it was not my heart but my lungs. I don't understand. Am I going to die? Am I going to leave the hospital? What is the prognosis, Doctor? What is the prognosis?"

"My name is Dr. Rosenblum," I said, deliberately speaking slowly. "Dr. Starch asked me to come."

"Good. Well, he must have told you what was wrong. I've got . . ."

His voice broke. I waited several seconds before he spoke again.

"I can't say it," he finally said.

"You've got lung cancer," I told him.

"That's what he told me, although I still can't quite believe it. You're a specialist. Can't you do something for me? I want to be cured. I've got a wife, grandchildren, a career. I'm only sixty-one years old. I've got to teach. I'm going to Warsaw in three weeks. Important people are expecting me. Their businesses depend on me."

His eyes darted about the room as if he were looking for a path of escape. He fired questions without waiting for replies. When I spoke, he looked befuddled, as if my answers increased his uncertainty. I felt as if I were a lifeguard fighting human terror as I tried to rescue a drowning man. Instead of identifying me as a friend who had come to help him, he fought me as if I were on the attack. He writhed with pain whenever I began to talk to him. My carefully chosen words explained nothing to him, provided no support. The more I said, the worse he seemed to feel. His nervousness made me uncomfortable, too. I wanted to escape.

"I want to review the X-rays, look at the slides, make certain I have all the facts before I talk with you," I said. "I'll come back Monday."

"Must I wait *that* long?" he asked. "I was hoping you would be back much sooner."

Time. I wanted more, he wanted less. I hoped the passage of time would enable him to absorb the shock of discovery so we could talk. His impatience was probably prompted by the pain of his anxiety, a feeling he may have believed would vanish if I said the right words. But the only words that would make his anxiety vanish were words I could not say.

"The time will be used well. Dr. Starch wants to use medicine to control the fluid. I can't do anything about your cancer until the tubes are out of your chest and you are back on your feet."

He did not relax.

"I want you to be able to reach me, Mr. Thompson," I said. "Here's my card. I will be out of the hospital during the weekend, but I've written my home telephone number on the card. If your questions can't wait until Monday, call me."

I wrote a brief note in his chart before I left.

Although a colleague had seen my patients during the weekend, I was not surprised when the telephone rang on Sunday evening.

"This is Julie James," an unfamiliar voice said. "I'm Mr. Thompson's daughter. I don't want you to see my father. He has had too many doctors in his room already. He is terrified. No one has told the family anything. My father is so frightened that he can't answer any of our questions."

From her tone of voice, I assumed I had been fired.

"What's happened since Friday?" I asked. My voice reflected no sense of rejection, only curiosity. As an oncologist, I have grown accustomed to being fired. Sometimes I learn the reasons; more often I don't.

"Some doctor told my father he was going to die and made my

mother sign a "Do Not Resuscitate" order. He wanted her to come to the hospital for a frank discussion with my father on Monday. One frank discussion will be more than enough for him. If he has two frank discussions, we are afraid he will lose his mind. He can't take it. He wants to live! All you doctors seem to want to do is to tell him he is going to die. He has been told his condition is hopeless. But he needs hope. I think he'll fall apart without it."

"I agree completely," I said. "In fact, I decided not to tell him much on Friday for just that reason. In the next week he will need to know a great deal about his cancer, but we do not need to rush the process."

Julie told me about the hectic hours of the weekend. She described the frightening possibilities one of the doctors had raised. At least a half-dozen doctors had seen him, several of them strangers. Toby had not understood much of what they had said.

"Those doctors were caring for his active problems," I said. "I'm not sure who they were, but none of them were oncologists."

"I understand," she said, "but he doesn't. He's never been sick before."

The previous Friday, after Dr. Starch and I had left, Toby's family had gathered around his bed. No one had spoken with them about his cancer. Not even his wife knew where the cancer had come from or where it had spread. No one had given her details about the dire prognosis.

"This thing's a mystery to us," Julie said. I could hear her sobbing.

"Are you familiar with anatomy?" I asked. "I have difficulty describing parts of the body over the telephone to people who are not familiar with it."

"No," she answered, "I'm a computer programmer. But my sister-in-law is a nurse. I'll get her on the line."

"I'm in pediatrics," the sister-in-law told me. "Take it easy on me."

"I think you'll understand everything I tell you," I said. "If you don't, you can ask questions."

I told her about Toby's cancer, the reasons for the hospitalization, and why surgery would not help him. I talked about treatment options. Our goal was to help Toby return home.

"Will he be able to go back to work?" she asked.

"I don't know. With hope, effort, prayer, and luck, many things are possible. Much depends on him."

"We've decided we would like to have you be Dad's doctor."

I had been fired and rehired in the space of forty minutes.

Finding Toby asleep when we arrived in the intensive care unit on Monday morning had been a boon for Ginny and me. I wanted to learn more about her husband before I talked with him. I hoped the details I could learn about his character would help me to be a better doctor for him.

When I arrived on the intensive care unit, I found her at the end of the hall, pacing in circles.

"Let's sit down," I said.

Nurses gently led us to a conference room and found chairs for us. They closed the door and poured fresh coffee. Although they remained silent, I felt comforted by their caring presence. I took a deep breath before I began.

"I feel strange talking to you," I said. "When I told Toby I wanted to talk to both of you, he asked me what good it would be to have you there. I don't know you, of course. Do you know why he might have said that?"

"He's the one who pays attention to details. He says I'm not organized enough."

"You'll have to learn. If he is still as anxious as he was on Friday, he won't be able to remember what he has been told."

"He's terribly afraid," she said, "but you don't know this man. He's the sort of person who can always handle everything. He always wants the facts. No matter how complex the problem has been, Toby has gathered the information and solved it. He's a specialist in management. He has an international reputation for solving tough problems.

"He's also athletic. He runs. He plays tennis. He's always active. Athletics are more than just exercise to him. I feel as if his vitality depends on them."

Her face tensed.

"Leave something of the man, doctor. Don't destroy him!"

"I agree, Mrs. Thompson," I said. "It would be wrong of me to treat his cancer and ignore his other needs."

She nodded her appreciation.

"So much has happened since Friday," she said. "He wanted to talk to me, to tell me everything. It was like going through the files and pulling out every folder. In one breath he told me he might die soon, in the next he talked about retirement plans. He jumped back and forth so quickly my head was spinning. One minute, he told me he was afraid he would not leave the hospital alive; the next, he talked about his plans for the next decade. If he died, he promised me I would not have to worry about myself. His pension might be gone, but he had plenty of life insurance. As if I were worried about life insurance at a time like this! I only want him to get well. I didn't care about the money. It won't buy more life. You see what my husband is like? I'm worried about his cancer, and he's worried about me. He wanted to be certain I had the key to the vault and knew where all the life insurance policies were located. He kept talking as if property and life insurance and keys and vaults had something to do with death. He didn't seem to understand I wanted him to live. Funny, isn't it, Doctor? Everybody knows about death; nobody's really prepared for it.

"We talked about all sorts of things, Doctor. I found myself saying things I had always been afraid to say. I told him I was sorry I was such a bitch. He said I wasn't a bitch. He said he liked the way I stood up for my beliefs. 'Intense' was the word he used to describe me. I laughed at him. ' "Bitch" says it better,' I said. 'I can never win an argument with you,' he told me. Then we both laughed. What is marriage, doctor? We've been together forty-one years and suddenly, like that"—she snapped her fingers—"it's all over."

"It's not all over yet," I said. "As long as you both are alive, you are still married. In the days ahead, your marriage will take on a deeper meaning than it has ever had."

She nodded.

"I need to know the facts," she told me. Her face looked deadly serious. "When is my husband going to die?"

"I don't know," I said. "I don't have enough information to predict the future. Some people with incurable lung cancer live more than ten years. Others live only a few weeks. Each person is different."

Then she asked me what and how I was going to tell Toby about his cancer.

As I left the room with Ginny, I felt a sense of familiarity and fear. My work has led me to have such conversations on a daily basis, conversations with strangers who are still reeling from the shock of discovery of cancer in their bodies. People who thought they were well one day and found they were fatally ill the next. Mine is a specialty given to serious conversation. Other physicians expect me to discuss sensitive issues with people I do not know, to talk about frightening facts without inflicting overwhelming damage. I wonder if anyone succeeds very often.

These conversations are the most difficult part of my work. In fact, much of the fear in such encounters has been my own. I try to look professional, to concentrate on my message, to put my patients at ease, but as I glance around the room, I see distress registering on the faces of the patients, the family members, the friends, and the nurses. I cannot forget that I, too, could be the person with the cancer or a family member or a friend watching a physician delivering a heavy message, telling the truth, even though it hurts, while I listen, helpless and impotent.

As a physician, tradition makes my feelings irrelevant to the task. The people gathered in the room, the patients and their families, have been burdened enough. Wise teachers taught me not to add my pain to theirs. As a responsible practitioner, I do my best to restrain my emotions.

But I have never liked cancer. I never saw any beauty in it. As a young doctor, I shied away from treating people with cancer. I hated pain, particularly pain I was unable to relieve. I wanted to treat diseases that could easily be cured. When I finished my residency, I considered the medical treatment of cancer to be hopeless. With confidence I told my wife she could be certain I would never be an oncologist.

An ironic twist caused me to change my mind. I decided to become a hematologist. I planned to do research in the biology of human white blood cells. I had responsibility for a laboratory, a technician, a fellow, and a research grant. As my work progressed, I began to publish technical papers.

Along with many others who began their careers as hematologists in that era, I discovered there were huge numbers of people with cancer in need of knowledgeable doctors and very few trained oncologists to fill the need. At the same time, hematologists had been trained in using chemotherapeutic drugs for what were known as "hematologic" malignancies, leukemia, lymphoma, and myeloma. As the budding field of oncology grew, hematologists were called upon to give similar agents to patients with breast cancer, ovarian cancer, childhood cancers, and a dozen others.

Hematologists who had been trained in major academic centers soon began to treat many kinds of cancers. Many took additional specialty training in the new field of oncology. Within a decade, the combined specialties were responsible for providing consultation services to a large portion of people with cancer. Before the sixties, physicians rarely turned to oncologists or hematologists for help. By the eighties, these specialists were often asked to see patients with newly diagnosed cancer. Because the surge in new technologies caused an expansion in the complexity of their tasks and the need for accuracy of diagnosis stimulated the development of exacting standards, such doctors became heavily burdened in their rapidly enlarging practices. I was one of them.

In practice, I maintained a strong interest in treating "the whole patient." I wanted to help the person with the problem in addition to treating the cancer. I made a pledge to myself to treat each of my patients with the respect I would want to receive if I myself had cancer.

In time, I learned to cope with my own emotions in order to help others cope with theirs. In the midst of sad situations, I tried to help people find a reason to smile. Although half of my patients would die from their cancers, half of them would be cured. I believed my patients expected me to find a cure if it were available and to help make life more bearable for them even if it weren't. I did not think they would want me to view the growth of their cancers as a personal failure, theirs or mine.

⊠

As we walked towards Toby's room together, it occurred to me that Ginny's questions were crucial: What *was* I going to say to Toby? How *was* I going to say it? For, rather than having a single answer to her question, I could think of many possibilities. I had no idea which one would work best for Toby.

Years ago, I used to have less doubt. When I was asked to see new patients, I would review the literature, extract pertinent facts from their records, and prepare an organized lecture. My presentation covered every relevant piece of information. All it lacked to make it perfect was a receptive audience. Unfortunately, I often noticed glazed eyes, digressive conversation, repetitious questions, anything but spellbound interest.

One day, a patient broke me of my habit of making such elaborate presentations. I had come to her with a polished recitation about her cancer. After a few minutes, she interrupted me.

"You look ridiculous," she said. "Your little patter is utterly boring. A handout would have been better, or do you think I am too dumb to read? I'll bet most of your patients forget what you say before you get out of the room.

"Concentrate on answering my questions. I'm intelligent enough to tell you what I want to know. I want to know whether

I can play tennis or if I should make my daughters have mammograms. I want to know whether I should eat more broccoli or have the water in my house tested for carcinogens."

Her advice was good. I decided to let my patients' questions guide me instead of insisting on delivering my weighty messages. The information was too much for me to communicate in a single session, anyway. I needed to experiment. I needed to probe, to find a method more suitable for the situation. But to do so would make me more uncomfortable than I already was. Without a prepared statement, I felt as naked as my patients.

Later, I was asked to see another patient, an elderly woman named Mollie. I spent an hour with her. She had recently been told she had breast cancer. A nurse had warned me about Mollie's fear. Although I had come prepared to answer dozens of questions about her cancer, I decided to let Mollie guide the conversation. She didn't ask any questions. Instead, she talked about her grandchildren and her work as a volunteer. She was deeply involved with her church and spent several hours each week delivering food for Meals on Wheels. She loved her work. With a twinkle in her eye, she told me details about the shut-ins she visited and how, upon being invited in, she often did much more than deliver food.

"Sometimes I almost feel like a doctor making a house call," she said. "I plan to continue my work."

I looked at my watch.

"I wish I could stay longer," I said. "I'm due back at the office in fifteen minutes."

"What a shame," Mollie said. "You've been such a dear to sit and listen to me talk like this. You must be a busy man. When you come back, I will have lots of questions for you."

I was offended by her assumption that I should make two visits to do the work I had intended to do in one. I thought my time was too valuable to be spent in idle chatter.

On the second visit, I found Mollie prepared for earnest business. Instead of appearing anxious, she had a keen interest in every aspect of her cancer care. She asked organized questions and seemed to understand the answers.

"You're such a kind doctor," she said. "You seem to understand what an old lady wants. I want to be myself. The things I do with my life are as important to me as practicing medicine is to you. When the surgeon told me I had cancer, I was more afraid of having someone take over my life than I was of dying. I want to be in control. The thought of having someone tell me what to do frightens me to death, Doctor, but I can see you will never, never tell me what to do."

Driving back to my office that afternoon, I felt a new sense of pleasure, a feeling that seemed almost out of place, considering I had just been talking with a patient about her cancer. My resentment about the second trip was gone. Indeed, despite the two trips, it had taken less time to talk to Mollie because I had not needed to repeat myself. Instead of expressing anxiety and confusion, she had been calm and receptive. As a result, I had not felt as if I were inflicting injury when I told Mollie bad news. In fact, we seemed to have made a mutual decision to face a difficult problem together. We had become allies. The first visit, for all its appearance of irrelevancy, had helped us develop a sense of rapport.

Had I learned enough to develop a "formula" for talking to people about cancer? For a while, I thought I had. I tried to imitate the method I had used with Mollie on a seventy-year-old man named Herb, a retired used-car salesman. Although he had developed a severe, incurable lung cancer, he was still chain-smoking cigarettes. My method was a disaster.

"Cut the crap, doctor," Herb said after about ten minutes of banter. "You don't have all day. As a matter of fact, I don't have a whole lot of time left, either. If I'm going to make every minute count, I don't want to waste them in chitchat. Just tell me about the cancer and skip the bullshit. We'll get along fine."

I must have looked disappointed because he added, "I mean no offense. I'm sure you are very charming. I've been around long enough to know who I can trust. Just tell me what to do and I'll do it."

He folded his arms and leaned back against his pillow while I gave him a prepared speech about lung cancer. He never interrupted to ask questions. When I was finished he shook my hand.

"Now that's what I needed to know!" he said. "Thank you, doctor, you were great!"

⊠

I thought about Mollie and Herb as I attempted to answer Ginny's question that Monday morning when we were about to go into Toby's room.

"I really don't know what I'm going to say," I told her. "It all depends on what he asks me."

Toby was wide awake by then. He was still picking at his breakfast as we entered his room.

"Where were you?" he asked, staring at Ginny and ignoring me. "I've been worried."

"You were asleep, honey," she said, giving him a peck on the cheek. "We didn't want to disturb you."

"I've come back as I promised," I added. "What do you want to know from me?"

"I need to make decisions," Toby said. "I've got a job. I've got a course to teach. What is my prognosis, Doctor? Am I going to live?"

"What do you mean?" I asked.

"Will I make it out of the hospital?" he asked.

"I think so," I said. "Of course, we can never count on anything. I suppose a piano could fall on your head, but I haven't seen that happen in years, now. You'll be home in a week."

"In a wheelchair?"

"On your feet."

"Will I jog again?"

"It's too soon to tell. If you try hard, even difficult things will be possible."

"What's going to happen next?"

I took a breath and sat down. Even though his bed was still raised and my head was at the level of his hip, I felt better than I did standing. I looked into his eyes, waiting for the moment when we would make a connection.

"Do you really want me to answer that question now?" I asked him.

"I think so."

"We both know that lung cancer is usually a fatal disease if it can't be cured by surgery," I said. "Surgery is certainly out of the question for you. But neither of us knows exactly what is going to happen to you or when."

I hesitated, waiting for him to ask me to be more precise. Toby seemed tired. He didn't ask a lot of questions. He seemed to be ready for me to leave after a few minutes, so I didn't stay too long. Outside his room, his wife asked several more questions. I answered all of them. I promised I would be back the following morning.

"If you need me in the meantime," I said, "don't hesitate to call. You've got the number."

In the evening, I received another call. Ginny wanted to know about Toby's medication. The conversation ended in three minutes. I felt as if we had become a team.

When I arrived at his bedside on Tuesday morning, I found Toby alone. His heart rate and breathing were much improved. Although his mouth was still dry, he was able to talk in sentences, to complete a conversation without constant digressions. I asked him to talk about his life. I expected him to tell me about the recent years. Instead he told me about an episode that occurred while he was a small child growing up in New York City. He had been less than two years old when he had the only other severe illness in his life. Members of his family had told him the story that meant so much to him.

"I almost died," Toby told me. "You can imagine what it was like. The east side of Manhattan, midtown, in the midst of the Great Depression. An immigrant family, all born in the old country. The whole family, a dozen or more, lived within a few blocks of one another. Nothing happened without everyone being involved. Children were precious to them. When I got pneumonia, they poured into the house. My aunts stayed through the night while my mother tried to nurse me back to health. They had no doctor, no antibiotics. I had a raging fever. Everyone hovered around. My mother wrapped me in blankets, my aunts made soup. I shook and trembled.

"My mother kneeled beside my bed, praying her heart out. She was a strict Catholic. More than devout. Her religion was as much a part of her as breathing. On her knees, she promised God that, if He would save me, she would walk barefoot with me in her arms to the shrine. When I recovered, she kept her promise. She carried me from our home on Seventy-Fourth Street and First Avenue to the Church of Our Lady of Mt. Carmel. It was forty-one blocks. She made the trip barefoot during mid-July." A warm glow suffused his face. He looked as if he had forgotten his fear of cancer as he remembered being nestled in his mother's arms.

I was swept up in the irony of his story. Toby had two severe illnesses in the course of his life, and both had affected his left lung. During the first, no medicine had been available to help him. Without the benefit of X-rays, tubes, biopsy needles, and expensive specialists, he had been cured by close parental attention and prayer. I wondered whether the modern world had a treatment as useful as the one he had received from his mother. Or whether, despite the progress of science, we could do no more for Toby than nurture him and pray.

As we spoke, I gathered the impression that Toby had been easily confused about his health problem because he had no experience in interpreting symptoms. His ability to exercise had become severely limited. He could no longer run. He was constantly short of breath, even going up a flight of stairs. But he thought his doctor had put a name on it. The doctor had told him he had bronchitis. The doctor had not told him what to expect, and Toby had not thought to ask.

"I was shocked when he told me I had cancer. It seemed crazy. For all those months I had assumed I had bronchitis. I kept thinking I needed cough medicine and lots of juice. I thought it would go away. I feel a little stupid now."

We looked at each other in silence for a moment.

"Cancer," he said, staring straight into my eye. "I'm think I'm getting used to it. I think I'm finally able to say I have cancer."

"Then it's time," I said.

"Time for what?"

"Time for me to talk about what we can do about it."

"Yes, I think it is."

"What would you like to know?" I asked.

For the next hour we talked about his choices. His mind was organized. His questions were pertinent. He seemed to remember what I said. Indeed, he focused on every word.

"Well," he said, when I had finished, "I may live ten weeks and I may live ten years or anything in between. I'm ready to get to work on it."

"I hope you do survive ten years," I said, "but your wife doesn't look strong enough to carry you from Bethesda to the National Shrine."

We both laughed.

And so we began our relationship, Toby and I. A week earlier we had been strangers, now we were linked by a disaster; we had banded together to work against a common enemy. Toby and I would know each other with an intimacy we would not have shared if cancer had not entered his life. We would share an openness that would have frightened people in good health. We would dare to ask questions that healthy people shun.

As we sought to link ourselves together, we would be reminded of the qualities of our personalities. Toby would come to understand me as something other than a generic entity, a specialist picked from a list. He would know me as a real person with a unique set of interests, strengths, and weaknesses. Similarly, I would come to know Toby as a unique individual with a special set of values, priorities, principles, and biases. For if I have discovered nothing else on the journeys I have taken with my patients, I have learned we are all different and cannot make ourselves fit comfortably into some preconceived mold. Rather than force ourselves to conform, we serve each other better when we learn to welcome the diversity that defines our place and person.

Down a dark path, beset by hazards, Toby and I would travel. Each of us would face personal risks more complex than the simple realities of cancer and death. The nature of our journey would be influenced by the baggage we brought along: our independent points of view, our personal needs, our faiths. We would sometimes find ourselves burdened by discrepancies in our points of view, conflicts between our personal needs, and challenges to our faith. Yet the success of our journey might one day be measured, not by its duration or its destination, but by the way we each listened when the other spoke, the peaceful solutions we found to our conflicts, and the trust we placed in one another.

2
VISITS

"IT'S DIFFERENT for you, Doctor," Ginny said to me as we were leaving Toby's room one day.

"What do you mean?" I asked.

"I mean the whole idea of cancer is frightening for me. I can't quite get it into my head that my husband has become a walking dead man. I feel as if the word *cancer* killed him even though he's still alive. He's not the man I married forty-one years ago. It's as if our roles have been reversed. I was always the chatterbox. Now, I can't say anything. I sit beside him, tongue-tied, feeling awkward. He was the strong, silent type. Now he talks constantly. I wish I could be like you, Doctor. You're used to it. It doesn't frighten you."

"How do you know how I feel?"

She thought a moment.

"I don't, of course."

"You think I'm not afraid because I've learned to hide my fear. I concentrate on other things, like the needs of my patients. When I'm sitting next to Toby, I try to respond to him and his feelings instead of thinking about my own. In the process of answering his questions, I forget my own emotions. His sensitivities guide my thoughts. His rhythms control my tempo.

"I keep thinking to myself, what can I say to buoy his optimism? I try to move us both out of misery to some happier place. Haven't you ever done anything like that?"

Ginny grinned.

"Not since I changed my baby's diapers."

"I have had more experiences with cancer than you have," I said. "But it is difficult to describe what I have learned from those experiences. I would like to make simple rules, but the issues are complex. I don't think anything about cancer is easy. The only thing we know for certain is that we are not certain about much.

"I've talked with several thousand patients. Many people have told me I am good at it. I try to be. But I feel best when I listen instead of talk. I'm constantly aware of my need to change with changing circumstances, to adapt to my patients' needs, to keep on learning and growing."

Toby was still anxious when I visited him the next day. He had a stream of questions, and he wanted them all answered immediately. I found him formulating a new question before he had heard the answer to the previous one, as if he were unable to listen or understand. His face betrayed his worried wonder, as if he were accustomed to taking responsibility for making decisions but lacked the background to be able to make judgments with confidence.

"Have you ever been out in a boat?" I asked.

"We have a day sailer. We often go out on the Chesapeake on weekends. When the wind is right, I don't know of a better place to spend an afternoon."

"I sail, too, Toby. I think docking is the hardest part of boating. I've spent more time learning the details, discussing minor points with my crw, learning to be calm and controlled while avoiding risks. We've never had an accident. But as many times as I've docked, if I were suddenly asked to dock a different boat, I would consider it a new challenge, one to be treated with respect.

"Decision making about cancer is far more complicated than

making decisions about warts, or hernias, or cataracts. In fact, if we were talking about boats, it would be like asking someone who had never handled anything larger than a rowboat to dock an ocean liner. Oncologists depend upon their interactions with other specialists. Despite our knowledge of the hazards, we proceed with extreme caution, ready to change our decisions when the evidence points in a new direction. I don't think you can expect to make decisions on your own."

Toby sighed and looked out of the window. For a while, he said nothing. I saw his shoulders droop. I felt regret about my comments, as if I had deflated him when I should have encouraged him to think about his problem with me. But something inside nagged me. I felt he was destroying himself by trying to do the impossible. He wanted to find a cure when I knew no cure could be found. Like others who are new to the disease, he had heard marvelous stories of people who recovered after doctors had told them they would die. Doctors had failed him in the past. How could he know whether he could trust me?

"I discussed your cancer with several other people," I said. "First at the weekly conference, then with members of the faculty at two cancer centers. The librarian provided me with a list of references."

I showed him several treatment plans. Later, our conversation turned to other interests. We talked about his family, his career, his interest in jogging. We joked about our frustrations with life. For a while we even forgot about Toby's cancer.

I started visiting people with cancer when I was in kindergarten. No one gave me lessons. I had never visited anyone who was sick, never seen the inside of a hospital. But cancer ran through my family like sprinters at the summer Olympics. My grandmother and one of my aunts had already died of cancer. Aunt Rose was to be the next.

My Aunt Rose was a tall, kind woman who had invited me to visit the family farm when I was about four. Her face had been as full of happiness as a sunny day, a happiness she had tried to share with me. A short time earlier, my father had been lost at sea, a victim of World War II. Aunt Rose sought to breathe some joy back into my soul. With a radiance that seemed to glow from deep within, her buoyant charm worked its effect on me. Tactfully, she avoided reminding me of my father's death.

Aunt Rose's delicate sweetness stood in contrast to my well-meaning but incautious Uncle Jake, who insisted on taking me into town to introduce me to my father's friends. My uncle walked me to the barbershop in the basement of the city hall.

"Here's Moe Jackson and Johnny Dixon," he said. "They were your father's buddies. Sam, the barber, used to cut his hair."

"I remember when I gave him his first haircut," Sam said. "He squirmed like an eel. Made out as if I were going to scalp him. He had one heck of a head of hair."

"Such a shame," Moe said, patting my head. "Your father was a wonderful man!"

I wanted to run away from the barbershop and the grown-up men. I did not understand what they meant by talking about my father as if he were a little boy. What did they know about the pain that penetrated deep within me, a pain they enlarged as they faintly echoed my monstrous grief? What comfort are the banalities of old men's talk for a heart so young?

With a rare sensitivity to a child's feelings, Aunt Rose had said nothing about my father. She had done her best to make each day of the visit happy by providing me with little treats and games. She made the kinds of food I loved and *never* forced me to eat vegetables. I smiled as I remembered the two weeks I had spent with her. She gave me a red tractor which soon became my favorite toy.

The following summer, I was taken to visit her in the hospital. I don't believe the adults in my small world understood what the encounter meant to me.

At first, I was not told Aunt Rose was a cancer patient. My mother had only said she was ill. As we prepared to leave, my mother knelt to tie my shoes. I could tell by her face that something was wrong. She had a sad, quiet look, as if she did not want to see Aunt Rose. I asked her what was wrong.

"Your Aunt Rose has cancer," she said. She whispered the word as if there were something wrong about saying "cancer" out loud. I had never heard her do that before.

"What is cancer?" I asked.

"Shh. I can't explain. Just get in the car," she said. "Your cousin Martin is going to take us to Johns Hopkins Hospital."

I sat between Martin and my mother on the drive to the hospital. Martin drove very fast. He had a cigar in his mouth that jutted up at a sharp angle. Although the front vents were open, the car was filled with the pungent aroma of cigar smoke. I hated the smell.

I listened while they talked about the war and President Truman. They did not say anything about Aunt Rose. They did not talk about cancer, either.

"Why do we have to visit her in a hospital?" I asked.

"To cheer her up."

"Is she sad?"

"Not exactly."

"Is she sick?"

"She's very sick. Your Aunt Rose is going to die, honey. She wants to see you before she dies. She loves you very much," my mother said. Out of the corner of my eye I could see Martin biting tightly on the cigar.

I had never seen a hospital. Until my mother told me Aunt Rose would die, I thought everyone got better when they were sick. I thought people died from old age or in wars, like my dad. I could not understand how my Aunt Rose, the vigorous, cheerful woman I had visited on the farm, was going to die from a disease.

Children were not allowed to visit the hospital, but Martin sneaked me up the back stairs.

"It's only a little rule," he said. "No one will mind. Especially if you are very quiet."

Aunt Rose lay in a hospital bed, propped up on pillows. She had brushed her hair and put on a bathrobe. She did not look sick at all.

I glanced around the room. No pictures hung on the pale green walls. A bulb in a glass globe dangled on a chain from high above my head. Light streamed through a huge, half-opened window. A fly buzzed noisily around the paper shade. I could feel a soft breeze bringing the summer heat into the room.

"Are you going to die?" I asked her.

Martin gasped. My mother put her hand on my shoulder.

"Not right now," Aunt Rose said, smiling.

"Good," I said. "Do you want to see my tractor?"

Aunt Rose laughed. Perhaps my mother had been wrong. We played for over an hour. Before I left, I told her I wanted to see her again, soon. But I never did. And when she died, no one told me.

During my early years as an oncologist, I sought to create a sense of enthusiasm when I visited new patients, especially if they had curable cancers. Like doctors in other specialties, I wanted to prove I was a success by saving lives.

In my first year of practice, my hopes of producing a cure were ignited when I was asked to see a man named Ben. At the age of thirty-five, Ben had developed testicular cancer. I had no idea what the disease meant to him. Perhaps, for one fleeting moment, my busy brain sympathized with the agonies Ben might have felt upon confronting the urgent requirement that he sign a consent to be surgically severed from one of his most precious and delicate body parts. If so, I "knew better" than to let Ben know I had any interest in exploring his feelings about castration. I was on a mission of much greater importance. Indeed, I had much exciting news for him. My hands and my awesome medical skills were going to cure him of cancer! I did not plan to reveal to Ben that my skills were derived from painstaking clinical studies done by others. To do so would have risked diluting some of the precious euphoria

I was feeling at the process of pouring a life-saving platinum compound into his veins. Only ten years earlier, I could remember watching young men die with testis cancer. Curative chemotherapy had not yet been devised. Sympathy? I had something more valuable. I had a cure. I was certain Ben would be delighted.

Bolstered by my enthusiasm, I hurried to Ben's bedside. The urgency was prompted by my own zeal, not Ben's needs. He was making an uneventful recovery from the surgical removal of his cancerous testis. Radiologic studies had confirmed spread of the disease to his chest. Several pathologists had examined the surgical specimens. All had agreed upon the diagnosis. The treatment I planned to recommend would not be started for several days. Ben had not been told about it.

Before I went to Ben's room, I talked to his family physician, who told me that Ben's life had not been a happy one. He had dropped out of school and struggled to find a steady line of work. For the past few years he had held odd jobs. He was currently unemployed. He had few friends. He had no medical insurance, and the costs of his surgery had forced him to borrow money from his parents.

The doctor had mentioned Ben's depression. "Finding out he had cancer hasn't improved his disposition," he said.

As I entered his room, I saw Ben slouching in bed behind a half-finished tray of food. A slice of gray meatloaf lay half drowned in viscid gravy surrounded by limp, yellow green spinach. He did not look up.

"I'm going to be your oncologist," I said. "Your doctor asked me to talk to you about giving you chemotherapy." At the time, I rarely talked *with* patients, despite my protestations that I cared about them. I talked *to* them.

He remained silent. Assuming he was interested in what I had to say, I continued to talk about the treatment I planned to recommend. I stopped, frequently, to interject hope and optimism.

"This is a curable cancer, Ben," I said. "Getting cancer is bad news, but if you are going to get cancer, it's best to get one we can cure. Get happy, Ben! You're going to make it."

I noticed a weary sadness about his face, a lack of luster in his eyes. I was afraid I had caused his distress. I did not ask him how. Although I was uneasy, I continued to talk about the treatment. In the midst of a detailed explanation, the door opened.

"You didn't knock," I said. My voice had an edge to it.

Ignoring my annoyance, a messenger, who wore a blue uniform with gold buttons, marched into the room. In a gloved hand, he held a dozen helium-filled balloons. They were brightly colored and metallic, the kind that stay inflated for days. One was shaped like a large red heart. Another bore the message "Get well soon."

"Excuse me," the messenger said, his face masked in a bland smile. He tied the balloons to the foot of Ben's bed and then handed him a greeting card. Ben dropped it unread on his nightstand. Without another word, the messenger left.

Guessing at causes of Ben's obvious unhappiness, I reemphasized the good news I had brought him. I promised him a high chance of cure. I offered to do everything in my power to curtail the side effects of chemotherapy. I described the personal attention he would receive. I felt as unsuccessful as a song-and-dance man performing at a wake. His face retained its impenetrable darkness. He grunted unintelligible replies to my questions. The harder I tried to please him, the more futile my efforts felt. I thought about his economic condition. Perhaps he was worried about expenses. The chemotherapy I planned to use would cost over two thousand dollars a month.

"If money is an issue," I said, "I don't want you to worry about it. I can make arrangements to get financial assistance to help provide your medications."

"Money!" he erupted. "You dare to talk of money at a time like this! Get out of here!"

"Perhaps this is not an ideal time to discuss your problem," I said. "I'll come back some other time."

Afterwards, as I sat at the nursing station composing my consultation note, I found it difficult to concentrate on my work. Ben's anger disturbed me.

"You can't please everyone," I said, half aloud.

"No," said an older nurse who was recording data across the desk from me, "but it never hurts to try."

"Trying has nothing to do with it!" I snapped. I was surprised at my own defensiveness. I told her what had happened. "I gave it everything I had," I added.

"Perhaps. But you didn't get around to the important part."

"What was that?"

"You never asked Ben if it was a good time to visit. You never asked him what he wanted to hear from you or if he wanted you to talk about his cancer today, tomorrow, or ever. You should have let him talk. You kept guessing how he felt, as if it were too much trouble for you to listen to him. Your style may work for some of your patients, but when people look sad and quiet the way Ben does, I've learned to be a lot more careful about how I talk to them. Ben was unhappy before he got cancer. He is not exactly having fun right now. Believe it or not, most people don't look forward to meeting you. It's not a lot of laughs for them. No matter how good you thought your message was, Doctor, he just wasn't ready to hear it."

"I suppose you're right," I said.

"I've had cancer myself," she said. "I know how my oncologist talked. He seemed to respond to me as a disease attached to a person instead of a person who happened to have a disease. I kept wanting to scream at him, 'Hey, it's me, Nan! Why don't you talk to me?' but I don't think he would have understood. He told me I was cured, but I never thanked him for it."

Ben fired me. He did not give an explanation, but his message seemed plain: he did not like my kind of help. I felt disappointed. I had lost a chance to cure a cancer. I can't remember feeling any concern about the reasons for Ben's displeasure. In fact, I probably thought he had foolishly misinterpreted my efforts to help him.

I was not fired often, but even occasional dismissals left their mark. One day over coffee, I complained to a surgeon about my frustration with "fickle" patients.

"Oncologists should expect to get fired," the older doctor told me. "There's so much anger associated with having cancer, it goes with the territory. People change oncologists the way they change clothes. When they don't like the way things are turning out, they go elsewhere. Don't take it personally. Some people are just difficult."

For a brief time, I was tempted to adopt his attitude. It provided a painless explanation for getting sacked. Anyone I failed to please was "difficult." I thought myself well rid of them when they left.

A retired clergyman wrote me a carefully worded letter. Not only had he fired me with good cause, he claimed, but my bedside manner could stand improvement. "It is a shame," he wrote,

> to see fine young doctors like yourself, experts in cancer care, who do not know how to talk to people. I wanted you to help me cope with my wife's illness. Instead, you filled my head with fears. I couldn't sleep. I couldn't push the awful things you described out of my mind.

I thought about his wife and the questions he had asked me when I discovered that her cancer had spread to both of her lungs. He had cornered me in the hall and begged me to describe the "worst thing that could happen to her." It had been an unusual request, but I had not stopped to ponder the strangeness of the question. Instead, I considered various possibilities, then chose to describe a condition that had frightened me. I wasn't sure it was the worst, but it certainly was a good candidate.

The Reverend became alarmed. I assured him I would do everything I could to prevent the situation. My reassurance had been to no avail. After our conversation, he brooded about the possibility that his wife would die a gruesome death. For several months before she died, he and his wife had been my most difficult patients. I had responded to daily telephone calls that dealt with each minute development in the progression of her disease. He came to me with long lists of imponderable questions. After I made it clear I could not answer them, he asked them all again, as if he had not understood. Tension clouded our relationship. I wanted to help the Reverend and his wife, but I found myself arguing defensively. At the end of a year, he fired me. A few days later, she died quietly in her sleep.

Six months after her funeral, the Reverend's letter had arrived. Without apology I responded:

> It is my policy to answer factual questions with facts. If you didn't want to know the worst thing that might happen to your wife, you should not have asked me. I try to be consistent. If you don't like my policy, you are free to choose another doctor.

At the time, I could not remember a patient with a more difficult husband.

There were ironies in our communications. The Reverend and I had been close friends before his wife's illness. I had saved his life when he had a heart attack. I had aided his rehabilitation by admonishing him to tailor his activities to the limitations of his injured heart. Many times he had expressed admiration for my careful explanations, my ready accessibility, my insight into his behavior.

When his wife became ill, however, he soon abandoned his grateful attitude. Instead of showing appreciation, he seemed distrustful, doubtful, unhappy with everything I did.

I was disappointed when he fired me, but not surprised. He had responded to my offers of help as if my best were never good enough. When I received his letter, I thought more than one of us could benefit from a sermon on behavior. Instead of respecting his thoughts as constructive criticism, I regarded them as the mouthings of an angry man. It did not occur to me that the Reverend might have wanted to be *helpful*.

Years later the Reverend's thoughtful words hit their mark. Time brought with it painful experiences that helped increase my sensitivity to people with tumultuous emotions. Personal frustration helped me hear distress and disappointment with a more practiced ear.

Time nurtured my growing awareness that beneath the skin we are all one when we are worried. We feel helpless when we have been bewildered by problems beyond our understanding, when we have been forced to cope despite paroxysms of fear. The orderliness of our lives dissolves in times of crisis.

"Coping is impossible!" our insides shout to us. Deafened, we hear little else. Isolated with our dear ones, we seek help from people who are supposed to care and are angry when they lecture us instead. When we ask questions, we want more than literal answers.

Caring physicians know gentleness beats accuracy when the questioner is anxious. They know people who ask clear questions could read textbooks if all they wanted were cold facts.

Time has not dimmed my memory of the Reverend's letter, his most valued gift to me. Although I glow when someone takes the time to thank me, angry letters are like manure on my garden: they make it possible for me to grow.

I decided not to label people "difficult." Calling patients difficult means that the needs of care givers takes precedence over the needs of patients. *Difficult patients* are excluded from the human family, exiled to a limbolike environment, because people who are expected to care about them feel overwhelmed by their problems.

Solving the complex problems of difficult patients has more to do with the art of medicine than antibiotics, chemotherapy, or calcium channel blockers.

A patient of mine named Lou described an episode in which he became a *difficult patient.* On one occasion, Lou was admitted to a hospital late in the night. No one on the staff knew him. A meticulous record keeper, Lou knew the name, dose, and purpose of each medication and was well versed on the treatments I had given him. He knew considerably more about his medical problems than the hospital staff.

39
VISITS

"You need to lie down!" a nurse admonished him when she found him sitting with his swollen legs dangling over the side of his bed. It was two o'clock in the morning.

Lou was gasping for breath. Instead of cooperating, he became angry.

"I don't *need* to do anything of the sort!" he croaked. "If I lie down, I'll die. I don't *need* to lie down. I don't *want* to lie down. If anyone has a *need* around here, it's you. You *need* to learn how to talk to people, if you *want* to be a better nurse."

Lou was right to refuse to lie down. If he had been compliant, if he had been as docile as the nurse might have wished, the fluid in his legs and abdomen would have shifted to his chest. He would have died within hours. Only by resisting her demands did he live to tell me his story about being a *difficult patient.*

When I probed into my relationships with patients and learned more about the effects their diseases had upon them and their families, I discovered that *difficult patients* were the most helpful in revealing the scope of the devastation cancer can cause in people's lives. *Difficult patients* told me many of the problems they were facing, not just the "relevant" symptoms of their illnesses. They told me about the subtle daily problems of surviving with cancer. Listening to them enabled me to uncover the vast, troubled world in which they lived. As a result, I, as their physician, could respond more effectively to their needs and, thanks to the insight they had given me, I could learn to look beneath the superficial, "satisfied" smiles of my compliant patients to catch a glimpse of their deeper needs.

Most people have hidden needs when severe illness strikes. Even the most confident people benefit from a sensitive visitor who is prepared to listen. Visitors who accept the burden of the difficult problems—the anger, the distrust, the confusion—give the people they are visiting a clear signal that they are able to share the burdens. Visitors who insist that patients be cheerful, put up a "good fight," and cope well place an even heavier burden upon them.

I also believe that all of us, laymen and professional health-care givers alike, should learn to make more effective visits to people with cancer. This year, more than one American will die of cancer every minute of every day. Whether we are patients, family, or care givers, cancer is a problem common to us all. It is better that we cease regarding cancer as bad luck or other people's problem and learn to cope with it.

A sensitive professional visit need not be undisciplined. As an oncologist, I never forget my important role of providing technical skill.* I must think of appropriate treatment as well as emotional concerns. I dare not ignore my role in diagnosis and treatment, simply because I care about human feelings.

Sondra helped put the issue into perspective. She was concerned she might have lymphoma. I examined her carefully. I could scarcely feel the minuscule nodules she described in her neck and groin.

"Don't you think I should have a biopsy?" she asked me.

"No surgeon could find those nodules if I can't feel them with my fingers. They're tiny. If they are malignant, they'll get bigger. We'll have lots of time to make a diagnosis. Haste would be harmful in this situation. I wouldn't worry about them."

I have never enabled anyone to cease worrying by giving this advice. Even myself.

"Don't tell me how to feel," she said. Her eyes blazed in resentment, then softened. "Your bedside manner could stand improvement, Doctor! Answer my questions, don't harp on my feelings about them. I don't have to hide my anxiety behind a pretty smile."

She flashed her teeth at me.

"Maybe your other patients hide their feelings from you. I'm not afraid to let you know about them," she said, "but my feelings are not the issue. I'm here because I have questions to ask."

*Unfortunately for people with cancer, a good many visitors forget their proper roles. When I am visiting someone who is *not* my patient, even though I am an oncologist, I do not offer advice unless I am asked for it.

I felt strange receiving instruction about my professional behavior from a patient. I wanted to tell her I did not need her help. But deep inside I knew she was right. As she spoke, I remembered a question I had asked a doctor years earlier. Instead of an answer he had offered me a tranquilizer. I wanted information, not drugs!

It was hard for me to understand Sondra. I began by trying to understand my own reactions to her. I thought about how I changed when I was with her. I became tense. I spoke in short sentences. I looked at my watch, counting the minutes until she left. Before I reconsidered my behavior, I had made other explanations for it. Now it became clear to me. In response to her anxiety, I had become anxious myself.

I overcame my anxiety by asking myself what it was I had feared: I countered my fears by taking steps to reduce the threats. I had been afraid I would lose control. I thought Sondra would try to take more time than I could spare. I thought I would become impatient with her endless lists of questions because I could not answer many of them. And what if she *did* develop a lymphoma? Would she be angry because I was wrong?

Knowing what I feared, I feared it less.

But although I was no longer afraid of Sondra, I was not certain I could respond to her needs. My anxiety improved. Hers did not seem to change. She returned several times with lists of questions, as if the answers I had given her had been forgotten or disbelieved.

"Why do you keep coming back to me?" I asked one day.

"Because you can admit you don't know. It's taken me a while, but I've decided I have no choice except to learn to live with uncertainty. Your willingness to accept your own doubts made it easier for me to accept mine."

In seeking to be a better doctor for Sondra, I accidentally learned something else. My success could not be measured by happy smiles.

I've visited several thousand people with cancer. I've had years to learn the art of medicine. And yet I am still uncertain what to say when people ask me about it. I want to help them, but for each of us the problem of speaking and hearing is different.

"I wish you could teach me how to talk to people with cancer," Owen said. "My brother is dying of cancer of the pancreas. Maybe you can help me. I don't know what to do. I'm about to visit him in Florida."

I was struck by the irony of the request. Owen was older than I. He had years of professional experience as a funeral director. He enjoyed a wide reputation for his sensitivity and concern. I was surprised he had asked me for help because I would have expected him to be safely guided by his own instinctive concern for others. Besides, I had never met his brother. How would I know what Owen should say to him?

"I'm on my way to the airport," Owen said. "You'll have to make it quick."

His anxious, weepy face signaled to me that he could not absorb more than a brief message. I wondered if I could condense twenty-five years of experience into a single word. Without thinking about it, I did.

"Listen," I said.

"Is that it?" he asked. His face relaxed by degrees. "Don't I have to ask questions, try to say the right things?"

"No," I said. "Trust your brother. He has the cancer. He probably knows he is going to die. I expect he will have things to tell you. He'll want you to listen, even though listening may be painful for you at first. If you are making the trip because you love him, listen well and your effort will be rewarded."

"Effort?" he asked.

"Listening is the hardest work I do. It is much harder than talking or thinking. It takes concentration. I have to let my own thoughts and feelings relax. My job is to respond to human needs. I must be comfortable with extreme intimacy, and at the same time, I must be restrained. My willingness to hear introduces me to a secret world within. I never forget I am a guest in that world. I tread lightly, ever aware of my potential to disrupt the delicate balance that constitutes a human mind. Yet at the same time, I can be a companion in the darkness. I stretch out my hand and wait for others to grasp it."

"I would run scared with your job," Owen said.

"I have to admit to feeling terrified at times. I have heard stories that made me want to flee. But I always asked myself how I could be of help. It kept my mind focused on the task. That is why I have come to believe listening well is the kindest thing you can do for your brother."

Owen looked at his watch. I could see he wanted to leave. I wondered if my advice would be helpful.

A week later he dropped in for a visit. I sensed an air of confidence in his step.

"Your advice worked perfectly," he told me. "I only wish you could have given it to the rest of my family. Mel, the brother who is dying, is the oldest. I also have three sisters and another brother. I tried to convince the others to let Mel do the talking, but they wouldn't pay any attention to me.

"I was real proud of Mel, though. He made a simple statement. He told us he had cancer and was going to die. He had been to the specialists, looked at all the reports. There wasn't any question about it. Everything possible had been done for him.

"My sister, Mary Jane, wouldn't accept it. She said if the doctors he had seen couldn't help him, she would find another doctor. No one should ever give up, she told him. She'd read about lots of cures. The important thing was to keep looking until you found what you wanted.

"Mel tried to be kind to her. He told her he knew it was painful, but it could not be avoided. He said he'd been to one of the best cancer centers in America. There was nothing left to do. He'd lived a full life and didn't feel like chasing after pipe dreams. He certainly wasn't interested in crackpot treatments that probably wouldn't work anyway.

"Mary Jane looked frustrated. She tried to find a place to send Mel for treatment, but after a while she gave up.

" 'I just hate to see you like this,' she told him.

" 'Don't worry about me, Mary Jane,' Mel said. 'I'm going to be all right.'

"Then Mel said he wanted to be buried in Florida. Mary Jane was dead set against it.

" 'Who do you think you are?' she asked. '*All* of our people are buried in Arlington. What right do you think you have to be buried in some godforsaken swamp? I think we ought to vote on it!'

"I said it was Mel's business where he got buried. He must have his own reasons for wanting to be buried in Florida. What does it matter to you? If it will give him some peace, let him be buried where he wants.

"The whole week we were down there, as long as the others were around, Mel rarely got to speak what was on his mind. You were right about him, though. Whenever we were alone, he poured out his heart to me, told me everything he'd been thinking about the family and his will and what he wanted done with his stuff. He told me about friends he had in the neighborhood, people who mattered to him, people none of the family knew about. After a while, he started getting into little details like the price of postage stamps and the fat content of salad dressing.

" 'Why are you talking about fat, Mel?' I asked him. 'You're going to die of cancer. Why bother with little details like that?'

" 'I'm still alive,' Mel said, 'and I have always worried about little details.' "

❖

It is easier for me to advise others to take time to hear than to follow my own advice. I know it is important, but I forget. My own anxiety and the anxiety of concerned onlookers sets my tongue in motion, as if an unending stream of words could protect me from the pain of hearing what might be hurtful to know.

When making rounds in the hospital, I like to identify problems and solve them on the spot. Occasionally I forget I am there to help people, not to *make* them feel better. When I *help* people, I take time to listen, obtain permission to work on a problem, make suggestions, and discuss alternatives. I let my patients stay in charge of the process. *Making* people feel better is arrogant. *Help* is almost always welcome.

One morning, full of the misguided zeal of a knight-errant bound on a crusade, I did not listen to my patient first when the nurses who were caring for him suggested I "do something" about his depression.

Ed was a fifty-five-year-old man with a rare form of cancer growing in his abdomen. The cancer, known as a sarcoma, had grown between the organs and spread to his liver before Ed realized he was sick. A surgeon had operated with the hope of curing Ed, but it was impossible. Certain his surgery would not help Ed, he ended the operation. I gave Ed chemotherapy to no avail. After we were convinced the treatment had failed, I admitted him to the hospital. Nothing had stemmed the growth of Ed's sarcoma.

Ed and I had developed a relationship based on frankness about his symptoms, his life expectancy, and the progress of his disease. Throughout the course of his illness, we had planned each treatment together. We had evaluated the results objectively. As a working professional, Ed had developed skills in managing administrative problems. He viewed his sarcoma as one more tough problem.

After he was admitted, one of the nurses told me that Ed looked as if he had lost all hope. She asked me if I was going to do something about Ed's severe depression.

"You look depressed, Ed," I told him. "Everyone notices your gloominess. We used to laugh with each other about your troubles but you don't seem able to dredge up a smile any more. I hate to see you this way. Perhaps you should talk to a psychiatrist."

"I don't need a psychiatrist to tell me how I feel. I *am* depressed," Ed said.

"Maybe a psychiatrist could help you with your depression," I told him.

"Look, Dr. Rosenblum," he said, "I don't mean to be disrespectful, but I have a right to be depressed. My wife died last year after a long miserable illness. I still grieve for her. In fact, grieving has almost erased my memory of the months during which I had to clean her, feed her, give her medicine, and stay awake with her through the night. She would have done the same for me, but she's gone now. Since she died, I have been alone. When I am in the hospital, no one visits me, no one pays the bills or looks after the house. I feel as if my life is out of control.

"You did not know about it, but my mother died last week. I was not surprised. She had suffered from several strokes and lived in a nursing home. Even so, I wanted to fly home to attend her funeral. Instead, you admitted me to the hospital. My brothers forgave me. They knew where I was. But I felt as if I should have stood beside them at the grave. I wanted to pitch a shovelful of dirt upon her coffin and say a prayer. I wanted to let her know I would be along soon.

"I hurt if I do anything except lie on my right side. I can't sit up, I can't care for myself, I can't even move my bowels without pain. The cancer has taken away my appetite. You and I both know the cancer is not responding to the treatment you have given me. Don't I have a right to be depressed?"

I felt the presence of the sadness in his life as I listened to him, a sadness that might have overwhelmed a man of lesser strength. But Ed did not cry. Instead, he spoke to me like an attorney arguing a case. Ed's longing for death sounded appropriate to me. As much as I had enjoyed laughing with him and breathing optimism into his fight against his cancer, I respected his feelings.

"I don't want anyone to cheer me up, right now," Ed said.

Listening to Ed, I felt much less like a doctor, much more like a personal friend. Rather than insist upon "managing" Ed's feelings because his unhappiness bothered *me*, I listened. I let him decide when and how he would seek to change himself. He was still sad when I left, and I carried some of his sadness with me, as, perhaps, some readers also will, even though they did not know Ed. But I felt I had been helpful, which eased my sadness more than I can say. I had given Ed time to grieve. I had been a witness to his pain instead of seeking ways to make him hide it.

47

VISITS

To my surprise, Ed looked brighter the next day when I returned. He even joked with me.

"We've got to stop meeting like this," he said.

"I keep wondering what a nice guy like you is doing in a place like this," I answered.

⊠

Caring people from many walks of life have shared their secrets.

"When I visit people with cancer, I never know what to say," a rabbi once told me. "Sometimes I just sit and hold hands."

"I recovered from cancer fifteen years ago," a bus driver told me. "I remember how much it meant to me when a visitor was willing to listen instead of trying to take my mind off it. I had a lot I wanted to say, and frankly, I wasn't too interested in what other people wanted to tell me."

Even my car radio brought me a valued lesson in visiting people with cancer. It was tuned to a music station. The announcer said he was in a downtown record store awaiting the arrival of Isaac Stern. Stern had agreed to speak briefly and then autograph a new release. But it was clear he had been delayed by several minutes. Impatient with the announcer's speculative chatter, I reached for the button to shift stations.

Before I did so, I heard Stern's breathless voice.

"I'm sorry to be late," he said. "I stopped to pay a visit to Hubert Humphrey. He's in the hospital again."

The public knew the senator had advanced cancer. In fact, radiation therapy and chemotherapy had failed to stem the growth of the malignancy, and it was known Humphrey would not live more than another year.

"I went to the hospital to cheer him up," Stern said. "Hubert cheered me up."

In a simple phrase, Stern revealed the nature of spontaneity between friends during what might otherwise have been a painful visit for them both. He had been able to listen, respond, laugh at Humphrey's jokes, find strength in Humphrey's optimism in the midst of a sad reality. Not only did Stern care for Humphrey,

Humphrey cared deeply for Stern. Cancer notwithstanding, the relationship endured. If Humphrey had been asked, I suspect he would have said that one of the worst burdens of his illness was the grief he knew it caused those who loved him. The violinist made an effective visit because he let Humphrey lead the way. Some of Humphrey's burden was lifted because he was permitted to relieve Stern's distress.

I thought about this episode months later when I heard the strains of Stern's violin in the Capitol rotunda where Humphrey lay in state. Of all the major political figures who have had cancer during the past generation, none surpassed Humphrey in courage and determination. He was committed to himself as well as to those he cared about, which was just about everybody.

The lessons I have learned about making visits to people with cancer are hardly new. Indeed, in the Book of Job, the ancients described the anger which well-meaning visitors can cause. I was never more aware of this than in my conversation with Maggie, an elderly woman who had advanced cancer and severe heart disease.

"My sister told me to read Job!" she said to me one day when I was visiting her in the hospital. She was too weak to get out of bed at the time. "She told me to stop complaining and read Job. Maybe I would learn to accept my troubles. She knows I'm a religious person. I wonder if *she* has read Job."

"What do you mean?" I asked.

"She said people always talk about the 'patience of Job.' I don't think they have read the book very carefully. Job believed in God. He went through a lot of personal suffering without complaint. He lost everything he owned. All of his children died. He accepted it. He prayed. He blessed the name of God. Then he became ill. Sores broke out all over his body. I don't know what they were, but they might as well have been cancer. No one could cure them. Still, Job refused to curse God."

"Maybe that's why people say he was patient."

"But he wasn't," Maggie said. "He had visitors who showered him with advice. They told Job he must have done something wrong to have suffered so much. They kept telling him to repent. They made it sound as if it were his fault he got sick. But Job knew he hadn't done anything wrong.

"Maybe you have to have cancer to understand it, but I think the wise men didn't understand Job. They never asked him how *he* felt. They never asked him what *he* thought had caused his suffering. They certainly didn't ask him what he was going to do about his problems and whether they could help him. They just told him how he could improve himself, as if they knew better than he did. No wonder Job got angry!

"I'm not a brilliant person, doctor. I never got beyond high school. I don't know much about medicine. I do know one thing, though. People don't understand what it is like to have cancer unless they have it."

"You are not the first person to tell me that, Maggie."

I went home and read Job, seeing the wisdom of Maggie's insight through new eyes. The wise men appeared to be interpreters of God's wisdom, people who assumed God is guided by human reason the way they imagined themselves to be. Job spurned their efforts. He wanted a direct confrontation with God. He cried out for justice, willing to bear the punishment if he could know his crime.

When he heard God's voice in the wind, the vast complexity of creation became apparent to him. Only when he saw his own smallness did he finally comprehend God's ways. For no deity worthy of responsibility for the entirety of creation could possibly change the course of the universe to satisfy a single individual's demands.

But just as God could not change the universe to improve Job's lot, He could not have altered Job's body as a punishment. Knowing his illness was not a punishment from God released Job from his need for justice.

When I returned to Maggie's room the next day, we discussed her medical problems. She mentioned her failing vision, her deafness, and shortness of breath. Her bladder had failed her so frequently she was forced to wear a diaper. Her bowels functioned only with the aid of medications and, even then, rather erratically. Her cancer extended across her chest and into her bones. She had survived many years with her illnesses, but her health problems had become insurmountable. She needed expensive assistance around the clock, and she had no money to pay for it.

"When I was a young woman I had a choice," she told me. "My husband became too ill to work. He had heart disease. We weren't wealthy. I had to choose between my own comfort and his. I never hesitated in making my decision. I spent all our money on him. I've been poor ever since. We had no children. The only one I could turn to was my sister, and she was not well herself. Life has been a constant struggle for me."

I listened to Maggie's problems, dutifully writing each one in the chart. I thought about the many treatments we had tried in the past, treatments that no longer seemed to help her. I found myself staring at my "progress" notes, unable to formulate a plan of action, unable to recommend treatment strategies that would relieve her symptoms. She had been seen by several consultants who also expressed a sense of helplessness.

"I want to do something for you," I said, "but as I listen to your problems, I can't think of anything I can do to help."

"And to top it all off," Maggie added, "I've been waiting all morning for some ice."

Then, because it was the one problem I knew I could solve, I took her pitcher to the ice machine and filled it. It made us both feel better.

3
HELP

And some kind of help is the kind of help
that helping's all about.
And some kind of help is the kind of help
we all can do without.*
—Shel Silverstein

A FEW weeks after Toby left the hospital, I received a call from Julie James.

"I hope you remember me, Dr. Rosenblum," she began.

I couldn't.

"I'm one of Toby Thompson's daughters," she said. "We want to help him."

I remembered her telephone call after my first visit to Toby. I wondered if they planned to "help" Toby by firing me again. I reviewed my management, searching for errors in communication. As far as I knew, Toby and Ginny felt comfortable with the care I was giving them.

"Has he given you permission to talk to me?" I asked.

"Is it necessary?"

*Shel Silverstein, "Helping," Ms. Foundation for Women, Inc. (1972).

"Absolutely," I said. "Aside from the legal issue, Toby's privacy should be under his own control. I'm happy to have a conference with you if he knows about it."

Toby granted permission without hesitation. A week later, his three daughters, Julie, Annie, and Billie, joined me in my office.

"I hope you don't mind if I eat a sandwich while we talk," I said. "I've given you my lunch hour."

My apparent ease contrasted with my inward tension. Although I have participated in many such discussions, I still feel like a general at a press conference. I expect people to want clear, precise answers to every question, even when clear, precise answers are inaccurate or wrong. I expect people to judge my competence by my answers, yet cancer treatment is too complex to describe in brief conversations.

I surveyed the three women. They would want more than knowledge from me. They would want to feel they understood what was happening to their father.

The three women looked unrelated to each other. Julie was dressed in attractive, friendly colors. Her warm smile reassured me. Annie wore a square-shouldered navy blue business suit. As she leaned back in her chair and covered her lower face with her hand, I felt the severity of her gaze. Billie wore leather fringes, beads, and long, loose hair that hung to her waist. She looked anxious and confused, as if any discussion of her father's illness was painful for her.

Their occupations matched their appearances. Julie was a social worker who worked with a hospice in another city. She was familiar with clinical terms. She told me she did not expect her father to survive. Annie, like her father, worked for a computer corporation as a program analyst. Billie, who had majored in art history, was "between jobs."

The three women fired questions at me as if I had just returned from leading the Union forces at the first battle of Bull Run. Aware that any comments I made might be fired back at me like hostile weapons, I spoke in measured cadences, choosing my phrases with almost visible deliberation. By speaking slowly, I hoped Toby's daughters would have time to consider my answers before jumping ahead.

"How may I help you?" I asked each one.

"Should we avoid giving him false hope?" Julie began. "You can see he's denying his illness. He's practically lost touch with reality. When his friends visit, he makes them kneel in front of icons. Dad was always religious, but he never prayed to icons. He always believed God was beyond human control. Shouldn't we make him understand what's happening? He should know he is going to die."

"What about a second opinion?" Annie asked. "I've read about cancer centers and experimental treatment programs. Hasn't there been a lot of progress? Aren't there thousands of people living today who have been cured of cancers that doctors thought were fatal? Why can't my dad try for a cure instead of quitting without making a decent fight? My dad's a fighter, Doctor. He's used to winning. Did you search the literature, call the cancer centers, ask the experts? It seems like every week I read about a new treatment in the Health section of the *Washington Post*. Why can't my father have one of those treatments?"

"He's not eating right," Billie said. "Can't we cure his cancer with special foods and supplements. Shouldn't he be on a special diet? No one has given him sound nutritional advice. Isn't that *your* job, Doctor? I've gotten several books about it, but I can't get Mom to listen. She's dead set on letting him eat whatever he wants. She doesn't seem to understand."

I laughed.

"Why are you laughing at us?" Julie asked.

"I'm not laughing at you. I'm laughing because I feel awkward," I said. "You each want to help. Yet you each see your father's problem so differently. An answer which would satisfy one of you might disappoint the other two. Yet each of you wants to help your father. Despite your differences, we all agree about our purpose for being here."

We spent an hour discussing the issues they had raised. I tried to fit their questions into the context of Toby's illness.

I thought Toby's behavior was his way of coping. We could measure his success by the degree to which he was able to function normally. He had remained orderly and organized. He cared for himself, talked about his problems, ate more, exercised when he could, gained weight and developed strength. He looked eager. He maintained his relationships with his family and friends. I regarded these as clear signs he was coping well.

"Toby never planned to have cancer," I said. "Like many of us, I think he believed vigorous exercise almost guaranteed good health. Unfortunately, none of the things we humans do *prevents* cancer. We can reduce our risks by avoiding carcinogens. But even if we do everything right, many of us will not escape.

"Every year a million Americans are diagnosed with cancer. Many of those people are young, vigorous, and healthy. Most people avoid thinking it might happen to them. It's too painful, and we want our lives to be painless. Perhaps Toby avoided thinking about the possibility that he might have cancer. What do you think?"

Julie shrugged. She could not account for the working of Toby's mind, his capacity to ignore what had been obvious.

"The shock of discovery of cancer undermined some of Toby's assumptions about life. He had faith in exercise. He believed he would never get sick if he ran five miles a day. Now he can barely walk a block. He needed a more reliable faith when exercise failed, so he turned to religion. He was not alone. Religious faith may not heal the body, but it can restore the spirit. To put it simply, Julie, I think he is doing his best to cope. If he is satisfied, who are we to judge?"

I turned towards Annie.

"We should make a reasonable effort to find a cure. You have raised good questions. In fact, I have asked myself similar questions because I am an oncologist. Curing cancer is my professional objective. I read constantly, attend conferences, and talk about problems with other oncologists. I also get lots of help from my patients and their families. Many of them bring articles for me to read. I have lists of references from the National Cancer Institute, the National Library of Medicine, and PDQ.*

"Before I made a recommendation about your dad's treatment, I reviewed all the information. There were many possibilities. But I had to make a decision. I couldn't do everything at once. I selected the best treatment I could find. I hope it works.

"I faced a dilemma shared by many other oncologists. No one has good answers to your questions.

"The best way to make progress is to answer questions systematically. Oncologists answer questions by means of cooperative clinical research projects. I tried to convince Toby to participate in a cancer study. It would have required time and effort on his part. He preferred conventional treatment. It was his choice.

"Before selecting a conventional treatment, I reviewed several recent articles on lung cancer. I discussed the details of Toby's problem at a cancer conference in the hospital. The other oncologists agreed with me. In three months we'll know if the chemotherapy has helped."

I paused a moment before I turned to Billie.

"I'm probably not going to do too well with the issues you raised. You've mentioned what I would call alternative forms of treatment. I have trouble with them. Most of the methods lack scientific proof. Before I say one method is more effective than another, I want to see a critical comparison. Anything else looks like speculation to me. But I do believe he should eat properly. The next time I see him, I will review his diet with him. I would be happy to send him to a nutritionist."

Annie tossed her hair over her shoulder, smiling.

"I expected you to say something like that," she said.

"I'm glad I didn't disappoint you. May I make a suggestion?"

"Of course," Julie said.

*Physician Data Query, an on-line data base designed by the National Cancer Institute to assist physicians in the treatment of cancer.

"Don't forget you are his daughters. As much as you want to help me do my job better, your job is even more important than mine. I am only his doctor. All I can do is to give him medical care. I know chemotherapy is adding to his burden. As his family, you can help him more than I. Your love is better therapy than my medications. In fact, even if it works, my chemotherapy probably will not help him for long. But unless I'm much mistaken, your attention cannot fail."

Each one gave me a hug before she left.

❖

After Toby's daughters departed, I could not avoid musing on the irony of my profession. As an oncologist, I have acquired much skill in helping people with cancer. As Toby's physician, I expected to use my skill to the best possible advantage. Yet his worried daughters, seeking ways to help their father, were more likely to help him than I would.

As I bit into an apple, I considered the sweet-sour incongruity of medicine's ideals and achievements. We strive to help; despite our efforts we often fail. Worse yet, our burdensome treatments may add to human suffering. We strive. With skill we strive, because truly helping one's fellow human beings makes other goals dwindle to insignificance. But, while the best way to help people may be clear to their families, it is often cloudy to professionals who devote their lives to healing. Because the path is difficult to find, we need to ask how we can be of help.

❖

No matter how much I want to help, I often feel frustrated in the attempt. Few cancers have frustrated me more than Jane's. Few patients have been as comforting.

Jane had an unusual form of breast cancer. She enjoyed seven disease-free years following her mastectomy before a sharp pain in her chest heralded a relapse. A bone scan confirmed our suspicions: the breast cancer had spread to her ribs.

57

HELP

"Is this inevitable?" Jane asked. "Does cancer always come back?"

"On the contrary," I said. "Breast cancer rarely returns after so many disease-free years."

We were philosophical. We both believed human life was more interesting because of the unusual events that build our characters. At times, both of us would have gladly sacrificed some character, if life had offered us a choice.

Although I sought to eradicate Jane's recurrent cancer, it proved to be resistant to every form of therapy. Jane's husband watched my efforts with a sense of resignation. But as fervently as I struggled to "help" Jane achieve remission of her cancer, nothing succeeded.

"Thank you for coming," I once said to Jane when she visited my office.

"Why did you thank me?" she asked. "I'm the one who should be thanking you."

"I'm thanking you for trusting me," I said. "Even when the treatments fail, you trust me. Such trust takes courage."

"It's not your fault the chemotherapy hasn't worked. All you can do is prescribe it. You can't breathe magic into it."

Her words were right. Her sentiment was right. I wanted to believe her. Yet I felt irritated and dissatisfied with my own helplessness. I never have been happy with the suffering caused by chemotherapy. At least, for those who attained remission, the suffering has had a purpose. For those who did not, however, the suffering was an unwelcome addition to the misery of having cancer.

Although I sometimes wish I could choose which patients would benefit from chemotherapy, I am grateful I can't. If I could select patients who "deserved" to be cured, the burden of making choices would be dreadful. I am glad I cannot choose the "lucky" ones by care or prayer. I'd rather leave it up to chance.

I often found myself balancing on a tightrope with Jane. She demanded the unvarnished truth, yet I could see how visibly clinical discussions accelerated her decline. I emphasized optimistic truths in order to sustain her in her struggle to persevere. Occasionally, she would sense my efforts to protect her.

"Let's face it," Jane would say. "I'm going to die of cancer. It's just a matter of time."

I didn't disagree. But if she knew she was going to die, what could my repetition add?

"We're all going to die," I said. "It's what we do with the life we have that makes the difference."

After she left, she wrote me a note.

> Once again you dragged me from the depths. You seem to know just what to say and when to say it.

My eyes stung as I read it. I did not feel worthy of such praise and admiration. As good as the warmth of her appreciation could have made me feel, it did nothing to take away the sting of anger at my inability to make her cancer vanish.

"How do I know what I should say?" I wondered, silently. "I want to treat her with respect, to honor her intelligence with honesty. But what is honesty? I never know whether what I consider to be facts will give her an accurate picture of her future. What does it mean to have a 20 percent chance of responding to a new treatment?"

Even though she thirsted for information, Jane did her best to respond to dark possibilities with optimism. She continued to work, though work exhausted her, because it provided distraction. Although her cancer had progressed, she continued to punctuate her weeks of work with happy interludes. She thirsted for life cycle events, for reunions, birthdays, weddings, and grandchildren. She longed for travel. Its increased difficulty did not dissuade her.

"I've always dreamed about traveling to Peru," she told me. "My husband wants to take me. Do you think I will survive the trip?"

"If you go up in the Andes, you will be taking a risk," I said. "Even people with normal lungs can have difficulty breathing at fifteen thousand feet. The cancer has invaded your lungs and left you short of breath. What will you do if you can't get enough oxygen?"

"Life is full of risks," she said. "Besides, I've been reading Mario Vargas Llosa's novels. I want to see Peru. I want to be a witness to the struggles he depicted. As miserable as my cancer is, it has come after years of productive life. There are large groups of people in Peru who spend their whole lives in agony. On my worst days, I have more hope than they do on their best days.

"Cancer is but one of the many serious problems we humans have to face. I want people to know I am concerned for them, not just for myself."

I did not want to give Jane permission to travel. I envisioned trouble at high altitudes, trouble that might be impossible to resolve because of a lack of medical facilities. But if I denied her request, I might destroy her dream. Because keeping dreams alive is as important to me as treating cancer, I let her go.

She loved the trip. She returned with two albums of photographs and scores of stories to tell. She described the majestic grandeur of the Andes, the dense wilderness inhabited by peoples whose mythic beliefs and ancient ways made Maryland seem like a settlement on a remote planet. She spoke of handmade implements, dirt floors, cockroaches everywhere, strange-looking foods, and dark eyes with impenetrable expressions.

"We call it the Third World because they have not become like us," she said. "But when I think of what our civilization has done with its portion of the planet, I wonder if becoming like us is such a good thing.

"You, too, should open your eyes. You should think about the broader problems of the world. Cancer is but one illness among many. I hope I never magnify my own needs and ignore everyone else's."

Early the following year, Jane could no longer leave her home. Weakness and painful bones made even short trips an ordeal. A team of nurses helped make certain she was comfortable. Although she was not in pain, she asked me to make a house call.

Determined to oblige her, I agreed to come. As I drove to her house, a light rain began to fall. Jane's street was lined with Japanese cherry trees in full blossom. Their delicate beauty contrasted with the serious nature of my trip.

I had been summoned for a final conversation, a farewell visit. Without being told, I knew I would never see Jane again. The rain grew heavier as I approached her house. A woman with a serene smile greeted me at the door. She was a nurse, sent by a local hospice. She had been with Jane almost daily.

A hospital bed had replaced the furniture in her living room. Jane looked restless, a jumble of sheets and covers was twisted around her body. Near her right shoulder, an intravenous stand reached two feet above her head. Suspended from one of its branches was a bag labeled Morphine. Tubing permitted the narcotic to flow into a permanent intravenous line. Although a casual observer might not have noticed it, one arm was a bit swollen. Her hair was thin. Her complexion had grayed. Beyond these few details, her appearance had changed little since the days before her relapse, three years earlier. Yet Jane and I both knew she had only weeks to live.

"What can I do to help you, Jane?" I asked.

"You came," she said. "That's what I wanted."

It was not the first time a homebound patient had told me about the powerful reassurance of a doctor's presence. I had nothing to add to the excellent care that her family, aides, and nurses had provided. Her husband asked a few questions about the medication, but he seemed able to judge his wife's needs. I listened while they talked about their grown children and their grandchildren. Jane had labeled boxes for each of them.

"There's a box for you on the hall table," she said. "Something I've wanted you to have."

I kissed her. Then I left with the gift-wrapped package under my arm. After dinner, I tore off the shimmering gold paper. It was a statue of five people in a joyful circle dance. As I pulled it out of the box, I saw a card wedged between their legs.

Through the years we have known each other, I have learned there are few things I could be certain about, few people I could count on, but I always knew that no matter what happened, I could count on you.

Love,
Jane

A few days later, word reached me. Jane was gone. I had placed the ring of dancers on a coffee table. In the evening I stared at it, lost in thought. We dance the hora to celebrate at births, bar mitzvahs, and weddings. All generations dance together. The young have achieved a degree of maturity when they join the ring. The infirm sit by the side when stiffened knees and hips have slowed them down. A time will come when I, too, will leave the ring. But as long as I can move my feet, I will continue to dance.

"May the sweet taste of joy dispel the bitterness of grief," Jane's sculpture said to me.

My wife and I attended her memorial service. It was a bright spring morning, full of hope and promise. A woman I did not know was introduced as Jane's best friend. With dry humor and a firm voice she eulogized their friendship.

"We did everything together, but we never agreed about anything. I'm a devout Catholic. She was an agnostic Jew. I am a rock-ribbed Republican. She was a knee-jerk liberal. I like flowery prints and Victorian furniture. She liked solid colors and Danish modern. Yet we loved each other as people rarely do, because we could confront each other without apology. We never failed to identify our differences. We argued with each other because it helped us to understand ourselves. We wasted no effort on self-pity or wishing our lives were better.

"I suppose, at heart, we were both realists. We had learned to take our knocks because we had no choice. We had our priorities in line. One weekend last year, Jane was forced to make a choice between going north when her father was admitted to a nursing home and going south to celebrate her son's graduation from law school. She had unflinching loyalty to both generations. We sat in her kitchen, drinking coffee and batting the issues around. She wanted to do the right thing. Certain either decision would be partly wrong, she finally decided to head south.

" 'My son and I have been very close,' she told me. 'Because of my cancer, he won't have many happy memories, but he has worked hard for his degree and deserves whatever I can give him. I'll try to make it up to Dad some other way.'

"Family and friendship came first with both of us. After all the coffee I drank in her house, I even got to liking Danish modern, but I still didn't care for Jimmy Carter."

"I want to be of help," I said, as if Janice had not heard me the first time. Janice's seeming indifference to my professional advice unnerved me. She seemed to be ignoring me, as if she thought her own attempts at medical decision making were better than mine, as if her gut feelings were more useful to her than my experienced judgment. In many ways, Janice was a strange young woman, a woman who refused to be reasonable about her breast cancer.

"I am a unique individual and I value my uniqueness. I want to go on being the person I always was," she replied.

"Good," I said. "I can't think of a better goal. But I think chemotherapy will give you a better chance of reaching it than 'gut feelings.' "

Janice had weathered a mastectomy and breast reconstruction before she came to me. She was thirty-eight, full of vitality, completely well except for her recent cancer surgery. But the little cancer had become like a monster in her eyes.

"The surgeon sought to cure you," I said. "He's a good surgeon, but there's more to breast cancer than meets the knife. I want to improve your chances of being cured. It's called adjuvant chemotherapy, medicine after the mastectomy. It has helped thousands of women."

But Janice had a different view of adjuvant chemotherapy. Before she found the cancer, she had always enjoyed good health.

She had been highly athletic. She taught aerobics classes. She danced and sang and swam and jogged.

"I don't want poisonous chemicals coursing through my veins," she said.

"Neither would I," I told her, "but if they could save my life, I think I would try them."

"But they might not work," she said.

"I know," I told her. "But they might. The side effects are not usually severe. Most people can live a normal life while they are taking adjuvant chemotherapy. Besides, what are a few months of nausea and hair loss compared to many years of life? A small price to pay, I think."

"Perhaps," Janice said wistfully. "But you never know for certain. I am a person, not a statistic. I want to stay away from medicines of all kinds as long as I can. I think I'll be healthier. I don't want chemotherapy."

I fought to overcome her resistance. Although at one time I had been reluctant to use adjuvant chemotherapy, I had long since become convinced of its efficacy. Huge studies, carefully done, had won me over. Because I believed her life could be saved, I pleaded with her to take it. I respected her right to decide, but I believed if she decided not to take chemotherapy, I had failed to present the facts clearly.

"I wonder if you understand the seriousness of this decision. Many people experience denial when they get cancer. They act as if they were immortal when, in fact, they could die from it."

"But I am not denying it. I know what can happen. I am no fool. I have a dreadful fear of chemotherapy. I have heard so many awful things about it. I've heard you say it probably won't hurt me, but I don't want to take the chance. I want to try to cure myself through exercise and good food and confidence in myself."

"And if your experiment fails . . ." I said.

"If it fails, I'll come back to you for chemotherapy."

"But it would be too late," I said. "If we wait until the cancer comes back, we won't be able to cure it."

"I understand," she said. "I understand you won't be able to cure me if I wait, but I'm not convinced you can cure me now. It all depends on whether I have cancer cells at all and, if I do, whether they are sensitive to chemotherapy. Since you don't know either of those things, I'd rather take my chances on my own. The statistics may be against me, but I don't care. It's the way I want to go. I have the right to choose."

My face must have reflected my disappointment.

"Please don't feel bad," Janice said quickly. "You're a good doctor and a fine teacher. I understand everything you've said. I know I'm not following your advice. But it's not your fault. I've always had a mind of my own. You helped me enormously. You gave me the reasons for taking chemotherapy, and you did it well. I've thought about the risks and benefits. It just doesn't appeal to me."

I insisted Janice return for another visit. I wanted a second chance to explain the treatment to her. I asked her to bring a friend. Once again, we reviewed her situation and the results of the clinical studies. She restated the information until I was convinced she had understood. She still did not want chemotherapy.

"I've always been a 'now' person, Doctor," she said, as she rose to leave. "Right now I feel fine. Who knows what tomorrow will bring?"

I was torn. Part of me wanted to endorse her decision. None of us can peer into the future and know what's best for ourselves or anyone else. It is foolish of me to think I am certain when I am only making an educated guess. Science never speaks with firmness about the future, its theories are based on data from the past. Part of me wanted to force her to take chemotherapy in the belief I could protect her from her cancer. I wanted to substitute my impartial judgment for her impassioned hunches. But I dared not take away Janice's right to self-determination. Our democracy guaranteed her the freedom to choose. Unless we are all free to make mistakes, we are not truly free.

For several years, Janice came to my office about every three months. She remained ebullient and optimistic. She brought me books about coping with cancer. She continued to teach aerobics, music, and dance. She sent me postcards when she traveled. For three years I wondered whether she had made the correct decision when she refused the treatment I had offered.

Life changed for Janice when a glancing blow from a heavy door made her chest ache for weeks. She asked for pain medication, but I found her ribs to be sensitive to a gentle touch. I insisted she have a bone scan. A few days later we were confronted with proof. Janice's cancer had returned.

I said nothing about her earlier refusal of chemotherapy. I did not want to add to her guilt. But my face must have revealed my thoughts.

"I know what you are thinking," she said. "But I made the decision, Dr. Rosenblum. I cannot redo the past."

She had painful recurrent cancer in several ribs. I arranged for her to receive radiation therapy. Her pain abated.

"You may feel well for years," I told her.

My prophecy proved false. Within a few months, she developed pain in other bones. She gave up dance and aerobics. She became a legal secretary. Work at a desk would spare her weakened skeleton.

"I love the work," she told me. "For the first time in my life, I've been asked to use all my intelligence to help solve complicated problems. The attorneys in the office have become dependent on me for help."

"Do you want to try chemotherapy now?" I asked.

"I'd rather not," she said. "I can stand the pain."

"But the chemotherapy might slow down the progression of the cancer."

"Because my life is so precious, I'd rather not waste it taking chemotherapy," she said.

"Even if it helped you? Even if you found that the side effects you fear so much were not as severe as you expected?"

"I am not curious enough to find out," she told me.

Her bland smile convinced me she had isolated herself behind a wall of denial. Fatal illness loomed on the horizon, yet she would not allow its shadow to cross her path. She deflected thoughts of aggressive intervention in favor of homeopathy and entertainment. The small risks of chemotherapy seemed greater to her than the major risks of fractured bones. Certain she needed to confront reality, I sent her to a psychiatric social worker.

"I'm not crazy," Janice told her. "Just opinionated."

Janice made no progress with the counselor. She revealed the sadness in her life but found no remedy for it. Janice had a dreadful fear of death at a young age. She did not want to die childless. She did not want to lose the chance to fulfill the dreams with which her head was bursting, but she could not find a way to make a reality of those dreams, despite her longing.

Whenever the social worker suggested chemotherapy might buy her precious time, Janice shook her head.

"I've read a lot about breast cancer," she said. "I understand what the treatment can do and what it can't do. What it can't do is cure me. It could add years to my life but not decades. Years don't matter to me enough to endure chemotherapy. It's decades I want, and I can't have them. So why bother?"

"I don't think I'm likely to change her mind," the social worker said. She sent Janice back to me.

I wanted to poke holes in Janice's reasoning, but behind her façade of "inappropriate" joviality, she had a solid argument. Treatment could not cure her; it could only delay progression of her cancer for several months. Once again, the choice was hers.

Her cancer was not kind to Janice. Over the next winter, I watched her body decay as the cancer spread through her bones, sparing her other organs. Her limber spine curled and twisted until she had shriveled to a child's height. She hobbled with a cane. She winced with the slightest movement. Yet she continued to smile.

"I know what you're thinking," she said. "But I'm only forty-three years old, and I'm still here and having a hell of a good time."

"What are you doing now?" I asked.

"I'm decorating boxes for department stores," she said. She showed me three elegant boxes covered with patterned fabric and decorated with lacy bows. "One is for your wife, the others are for your nurses."

I held the boxes in my hands and examined them carefully. The handwork was meticulously finished, the colors and design of the print well suited to the shape of the box. Janice had turned a simple handcraft into a work of art.

"They're on back order at Saks and Lord & Taylor's," she giggled. "I can't make them fast enough to keep up with the demand. I should have been an entrepreneur."

"You should have taught a course in coping," I said. "I'm pleased to see how well you do."

"The pain has found a new place to lodge," she told me, using a ruler to point to the center of her back.

An MRI showed an ominous metastasis, a cancerous growth in her vertebral canal that threatened to crush her spinal cord. Although she had walked into my office, I rushed her to the hospital. Delay of a few hours might have spelled disaster for her nervous system. She could be paralyzed from her waist down. A neurosurgeon and an orthopedist assisted me. Together, and with Janice's consent, they undertook a lengthy operation in order to reconstruct two vertebrae that had collapsed. We both were thrilled when she took her first step. The pain remained fierce, despite strong medication, but she smiled bravely.

"I'm going to make it," she said.

Her happiness was short-lived. Within two months the cancer had reappeared in her liver. Janice greeted the news with equanimity.

"I guess it's time to try chemotherapy," she said.

I smiled wryly.

"You probably think I waited much too long," she told me, "but I haven't any regrets. Having cancer is bad enough. Letting chemotherapy dominate my life would have been worse. I've got nothing to lose now."

By some curious twist of circumstance, chemotherapy never affected Janice much. Except for hair loss, it neither made her sick nor caused her cancerous metastases to shrink. When she became too weak to get out of bed, she decided to return to her mother's home a thousand miles away. Weeks later, I received a note from her.

"I want you to know how grateful I am," she wrote. "I know I refused to take the treatment you thought would help me. I often argued with you instead of letting you be the judge. It's possible I made some mistakes along the way. It was important that they were *my* mistakes. Whatever consequences I suffered were the results of my own decisions. It has been my life to the very end. And now that death is approaching (and I realize that it *most certainly is*) I do not dread it as I once did. I shall miss my friends and they shall miss me. I won't get to do all those projects I once dreamed about. But I shall no longer have to suffer with this crummy cancer."

I do not know if I ever helped Janice but I know she helped me.

Janice made me think about my goals as an oncologist. Given a choice, I would rather "help" people than "treat" their cancers. Although Janice had exercised her right to choose not to follow textbook prescriptions, she still wanted medical advice. Rather than adapting her life to fit my medical recommendations, she made me adapt my medical recommendations to her life. My task was more confusing because the goals were sometimes obscure, but Janice remained in control.

"Chemotherapy is not for everyone," Janice once told me. "People can understand what it does. We're not stupid. Some of us want it because they'll do anything to stay alive. Others are more attracted by less confining choices."

Janice had been allowed her choices, as had I. For, in the best traditions of medicine, I had cleaved to the spirit of my profession. I had "listened to my patient" instead of insisting on the more common methods of treatment.

A poem comes to mind, a poem about choices and the human condition.

Two roads diverged in a yellow wood,
And sorry I could not travel both
And be one traveler, long I stood
And looked down one as far as I could
To where it bent in the undergrowth;

Then took the other, as just as fair,
And having perhaps the better claim,
Because it was grassy and wanted wear;
Though as for that, the passing there
Had worn them really about the same,

And both that morning equally lay
In leaves no step had trodden black.
Oh, I kept the first for another day!
Yet knowing how way leads on to way,
I doubted if I should ever come back.

I shall be telling this with a sigh
Somewhere ages and ages hence:
Two roads diverged in a wood, and I—
I took the one less traveled by,
And that has made all the difference.*

We cannot help without being willing to take time to listen and to hear. To listen best to people, I try to forget who I am and consider who they are, how they see themselves, how they picture their own needs. A woman I know named Alice described the process with sensitivity. The situation arose in a local grocery store. An elderly woman was shopping from a wheelchair.

"Would you mind helping me?" the woman asked as Alice passed her.

"Gladly," Alice replied. "What would you like me to do for you?"

"Please put a small basket in my lap and give me eight plastic bags."

*Robert Frost, "The Road Not Taken" (1915).

"Do you want me to pick out some fruit or vegetables for you?"

"That I can do myself, thank you."

"I would have been happy to do it for her," Alice told me later, "but she wanted to do it herself. If I had insisted on picking things out for her, she would have felt defeated. I felt the same way when I got cancer."

"What do you mean?"

"I have three close friends. We have gone through many experiences together. We graduated from high school in the same class, twenty-five years ago. We play tennis twice a week. We shop together. We've even shared vacations. We've always shared tough times as well as fun.

"When I got breast cancer, I wanted them to know everything about it. But after I told them about my mastectomy, our relationship turned topsy-turvy. They seemed to forget I had my *breast* removed, not my *brain*. Just because I have cancer doesn't mean I'm a mental cripple."

"What do you mean?"

"One of them clipped articles from newspapers and magazines. A second called the National Library of Medicine and started doing literature searches. The third one brought me "health foods" and books about nutrition. They bombarded me with information and advice, as if I were too stupid to figure things out on my own.

"Whenever I wanted to talk about a visit I had made to your office, they wanted to hold a group discussion to critique your advice. They compared what you said to the articles they had read or to things they had heard from other patients. I felt helpless. I wanted their friendship. I needed it more than ever. But their advice was making it more difficult for me to think clearly.

"They couldn't understand why I wasn't grateful for their contributions. But I didn't want advice from them. I didn't think they knew enough to give me good advice. They were only guessing. Guessing isn't good enough when you're talking about cancer. They aren't oncologists. They aren't even doctors."

"You're like the lady in the wheelchair," I said. "You weren't helpless, and you didn't want to be treated that way. Did your friends ask what you wanted them to do?"

"I wish they had," Alice said. "But until I got cancer, I would not have known how important it is to ask."

"My husband has lost a lot of weight," Doris told me. "He's dangerously malnourished. Isn't there something I can do about it?"

"I agree with you. Kevin has lost weight," I said. "But you can't make him gain it back."

"What about vitamins or supplements or hyperalimentation? You aren't giving up on him, are you?"

Doris was a nutritionist. She enjoyed a reputation in the community for her intelligent meal planning as well as her culinary skills. She conducted annual classes in food preparation both for the American Heart Association and for the American Cancer Society.

"If you eat right, it will help you stay healthy" had been her recurrent theme. Yet she knew better than to blame her husband's cancer on dietary lapses. "No matter what you do," she told me, "there are no guarantees."

Kevin was a concert violinist. He had a highly prized collection of baroque instruments. Each spring he took pride in presenting an evening of chamber music to fund a scholarship to send a few students to music camp. Over the years some of his protégés had become professional musicians.

When I told him about his cancer, he was not surprised. For weeks he had been fatigued. He had a gnawing feeling in his gut. And nothing he ate appealed to him. He had pulled his belt three notches tighter before he came to me.

"I'm sixty-three," he said. "Many of my friends have had cancer. I know it happens."

When Kevin's cancer was discovered, Doris searched the library for articles about replacement diets for people with cancer. Kevin's appearance trumpeted the reason for her concern. He looked as if he had been starving instead of dining at her well-furnished table.

We discussed the findings together. Clinical evidence had proven beyond a doubt that Kevin's cancer was far advanced. Blood tests showed clear signs of metabolic failure. Marker enzymes were elevated and his albumin was low. A CAT scan showed a large mass in his pancreas and multiple small ones in his liver. A needle biopsy had established the diagnosis: adenocarcinoma of the pancreas. We could make no appeal against the established facts. At best, Kevin would survive six months, but a shorter span was far more likely.

Doris knew I was powerless to change the course of Kevin's illness, which, like a death sentence, hung over him with grim finality. I knew of no effective treatment for widespread pancreatic cancer.

Doris and I addressed Kevin's comfort, skin care, pain medications, and control of his bodily functions. To make his life easier, she put hospital equipment in their home. She installed a portable telephone. She hired an aide to be with him when she was away. But Kevin's appearance continued to frustrate her.

"He looks bad," she repeated every time I saw her.

"But he doesn't feel bad," I said. "I know you want to help him. . . ." Her worried face made me pause. Who could look at Kevin and not want to do something? His gaunt face alone seemed to give incontrovertible evidence of need for food. My years in medicine had not erased my desire to nourish him, but I knew nothing we could do was likely to improve Kevin's appearance.

Destruction of his pancreas by the cancer might have removed the enzymes that were needed to digest his food. But even after we supplied the enzymes, he continued to lose weight. Liver damage limited his metabolism. Supplements, by mouth or vein, were of little use to him.

Kevin continued to languish. We wanted to help him, yet we could not translate our yearning into effective action.

"I know it hurts," I said. "Watching someone you love change into a specter of himself is like living through a nightmare. But we have to distinguish between our pain and Kevin's needs. He doesn't want more food. In fact, he can't stand the sight of it. It is better to let his body adjust to the cancer, no matter how painful it is to watch, than to appease our own feelings by forcing food on him. Keep asking him what he wants. Let his answers guide you."

After he died, Doris wrote a thoughtful note. Following our conversation, she had encouraged Kevin to express his wishes. Food and physical appearance, he insisted, were utterly unimportant to him. Instead, he talked about establishing an endowed scholarship for young musicians. He wanted to sell his collection of instruments. Through contacts in the community, he found appropriate buyers. Doris did the leg work because Kevin was too weak. She found an attorney to create the endowment. But it was Kevin's project all the way. She wrote:

"I wish I had learned to sort things out earlier. I needed to listen more. After I heard him clearly, I was grateful to have an opportunity to work on Kevin's goals with him. It was much less frustrating than making him eat."

"They say patients have to accommodate to doctors' schedules," Ray told me. "I understand what they mean. But when you're the patient, somehow it looks a little different."

"I'm sorry I kept you waiting," I said. "I couldn't avoid it."

"I know you couldn't," Ray said. "You're late because you've been helping people all afternoon. Whenever they ask you a question, you try to answer it. If they want more time, you give it to them. I know all this, and yet I'm still annoyed. Not with you, Doctor. Just with having to wait."

Ray was forty-five. He had three children under twelve. He also had lymphoma. He said the children were precious to him and the lymphoma threatened his ability to watch them grow. Children meant more to him than professional success. The simple dimensions of time and space acquired new significance after the children were born.

"I love life-cycle events, Dan," he told me. "I used to scoff at sentimentality. I hated ceremonies. I didn't even attend my college graduation. Now I thrill at graduations and weddings, even if I don't know the people well. I even love Father's Day and Valentine's Day."

Each year, Ray knew he had a 5 percent chance of dying from his lymphoma. Slim, but real. With each birthday, the likelihood of surviving another decade shrank perceptibly. Although he looked and felt well, worked full-time, and led a vigorous life, he wanted to improve the odds of reaching his children's weddings and graduations.

"How much time do I have?" he asked his first oncologist.

"Ten years, maybe. If you're lucky, you could live fifteen or twenty," the doctor had said.

" 'Could,' you say?"

"There's no way of telling who will survive the longest."

Too sensible to complain, Ray lived under the shadow of an imaginary clock ticking the months away, a constant reminder of the inestimable value of each moment.

He never lost his flair for bench research. In fact, he felt his thoughts of death sneak away into a dark corner when he labored, late at night, on an obscure problem. At home, wrapped up with the life of his family, he could easily forget the tiny nodes in his neck and groin, lumps which spelled a future he preferred to forget.

But in the quiet times, his equanimity seemed as fragile as spun glass, ready to shatter if he breathed the words "how long?" The quiet times arrived without announcement. Occasionally, he would be hard at work, absorbed in solving a complex problem in the laboratory, yet when he looked up from his notebook and saw the Christmas photograph of his family, he would shudder. At such times he would wonder if the children perched on his knees would have no knees to sit on when the next Christmas arrived. During one such moment, he noticed his son was holding two fingers in a V behind his head. He laughed. He had mailed fifty pictures of himself playing the jackass to a six-year-old. But even his laughter was cut short when he realized he might not have a chance to laugh at such a prank again.

He told his oncologist about his fears, and his oncologist responded by ordering a series of tests.

"They told me the tests would help me, but they never told me how," he said. "In fact, they never told me much at all."

I knew Ray had fired his first oncologist before he came to me. I did not know why.

"It isn't what you think," he said. "You think I have complicated ideas. You imagine I have scoured the medical journals looking for curative treatments. Wrong. It wasn't anything like that. Perhaps I shouldn't tell you."

"I don't mind listening if you want to talk."

"I shouldn't complain," Ray said. "I know doctors aren't perfect. I understand they are human. They make mistakes. I try not to exaggerate."

"And I accept your view. What happened?"

"They wanted to do a liver biopsy. I expected it to be done in the morning. No one told me the doctor would be away until evening. He did not start the procedure until nine o'clock that night. The anesthesiologist was young. I did not think he knew what he was doing. It was July. The interns and residents were still quite new at their jobs.

"The doctor made a small incision in my abdomen and inserted an instrument. I was supposed to be asleep, but midway through the procedure I woke up. I was groggy, confused. I thought I was somewhere else. I felt someone kicking me in the side. I sat up. I tried to get away. The instrument came out. I remember yelling at them. Then, suddenly, I was asleep again. I didn't remember anything until I woke up.

"The doctor never apologized for the accident. He never said a word about the inadequate anesthesia. He seemed to be worried about the damage I might have caused when I sat up. He did not seem to know I had been confused, groggy, frightened, and out of control. He said the instrument might have poked a hole in my intestine.

" 'You certainly made a lot of trouble for us," he said. 'You should never move around with an instrument inside of you.'

"They put me in the intensive care unit. I lay there for hours with nurses taking frequent vital signs. I did not know what they expected to find.

"At midnight, the doctor ordered a CAT scan. The nurses complained about taking me down to the radiology department. It was the end of their shift. They said they were tired and wanted to go home.

"After the CAT scan, I was left on a stretcher in the hallway inside the X-ray department. The air conditioner was blowing constantly. I was shivering from the cold. I had no blanket. I didn't know what the CAT scan showed. Nobody talked to me. It was after one in the morning. I didn't know whether I was going back to the intensive care unit, the operating room, or the morgue, whether my gut was perforated or whole, whether I had a fatal wound or there was nothing seriously wrong with me. Nothing serious except the lymphoma.

"Someone finally wheeled me back to the intensive care unit, but no one told me what the CAT scan showed. I did not hear about it until the next morning.

" 'We didn't see anything to worry about,' the doctor told me.

" 'Why wouldn't you tell me last night?'

"He never answered me. For eight hours, I felt as if my life were hanging in the balance and no one knew or cared how I felt about it.

"It's over now, but I never trusted the hospital again. I distrusted everyone and everything. My doctor asked me to call him at the hospital. But when I called the oncology clinic, I was told there was no doctor by that name.

" 'But he's my doctor!' I insisted.

" 'You must be mistaken,' she replied.

"She never admitted she could be mistaken," Ray said. "Even after she turned out to be wrong."

As Ray's doctor I wanted to heal his injuries and restore his confidence in the medical system. From his tendency to describe his experience in minute detail, I guessed at the pain he still felt when he thought about it. He winced as he described the twist of the instrument in his abdomen.

Together, we planned to arrange a bone marrow transplant. Studies suggested it might give lasting remission of his lymphoma. The procedure was risky, but encouraging results justified the risks.

Ray would meet new doctors, and would need help with communication. It would be important for me to help him avoid delays, mistakes, and miscommunication.

"I'll lose my hair, of course, and they mentioned a dozen other side effects. Besides, there's a 10 percent chance of death from bone marrow transplantation," he told me with stony coldness. "Maybe fifteen."

He laughed. The sound was short and hollow. And false. Death from lymphoma might not be as miserable as death from marrow transplantation. Death from transplantation could be due to human error, a possibility which had more than casual significance for Ray.

"Everything we do can fail," I said. "Airplanes fall apart in midair. Bridges collapse. Buildings catch fire. I can't guarantee to make the transplantation successful, but I'll ride shotgun for you."

The transplantation worked. He had no serious problems, although he suffered minor symptoms along the way. Tests performed at the university confirmed the likelihood of cure. Throughout the months of treatment, we communicated regularly. All Ray's questions were answered. His insecurity was eased by attentive physicians and nurses. When he had doubts, he had my telephone number.

"The system can fail," he said, smiling. "But it can also work. I could not have asked for better care."

At Christmas, when he sat for the family portrait, his children made him wear a fluffy white moustache and beard, a droll counterpoint to his bald head. He showed me the picture.

"I guess the process of making me look silly is going to become a family institution," Ray said with a laugh.

4
RELATIONSHIPS

Yesterday, we had not met.
Today, we two are one,
Linked by bonds we won't forget
Until we both are gone.

"I DON'T mind saying I have cancer. But I don't feel ready to call myself a cancer patient," Toby told me.

"Then don't," I said. "I like 'Toby Thompson' a whole lot better than 'cancer patient.' It tells me you're a person worth knowing instead of a disease underneath a hospital gown. Why call yourself a cancer patient if you don't have to?"

"But I *am* a cancer patient," Toby said. He looked at me quizzically.

"I'm not just playing word games," I said. "I think labels are dangerous. They force a mind-set on people. If you call yourself a cancer patient, you become a case of a disease instead of a person. Cases are dots on a graph. Individuals have character. Cases are charts with progress notes, laboratory data, and pathology reports. People are connected with the rest of the world. Your cancer is a tiny part of you. Your personality didn't vanish because of a few flawed cells.

"I never thought of it that way," Toby said.

"If you label yourself a cancer patient, it can poison your life. It divides you from the rest of humanity, forces you into a sort of purgatory. You run the risk of becoming what no one wants to be: an object of pity. They'll drop in and say things like 'Isn't it a shame?' or 'I was *so* sorry when I heard the news.' "

"What should they say?"

"What would you like them to say, Toby?"

He thought for several minutes before he answered.

"I liked what Lanny did the best," he said. "Lanny and I have been friends since we were teenagers. We were the sort of friends who could read each other's faces at a glance. When one of us was in trouble, the other one always cared. We graduated from City College in the same class. We were both *real* Dodgers fans. The kind who grieved when the Bums left Brooklyn.

"When Lanny heard I had cancer, he came rushing to the hospital. He left an important meeting and a busy day in the office. When he reached my room, he didn't say anything. He just gave me a big hug. It was a big emotional moment for both of us. I didn't want his pity, and he didn't give me any.

"When Lanny asked me what was happening, I didn't feel he was prying. He listened while I told him what the doctor had said. He didn't grill me with questions or make suggestions. He just listened. It felt wonderful to know he cared. Even now, Lanny never tells me what to do. He never gives me advice unless I ask for it. It's great to have a true friend.

"Jill, on the other hand, made me feel awful. Neither Ginny nor I knew her too well before I got cancer. She is the wife of one of my coworkers in the office. Without being asked, she started making suggestions on day one. She began with phrases like 'Your doctor may not believe this, but . . . ' and then she would give me some tripe about a bizarre treatment with coffee enemas and herbal teas. She never waited to be asked whether I wanted to hear what she had to say. I wish I could find a way to make her stop. My wife and I are both upset by her prating, but we don't know how to turn her off."

"Remember who you are, Toby. You're a supremely competent consultant. People pay you well for your advice because you do not give an opinion without checking carefully into the facts. Suppose someone with no experience appeared on the scene while you were giving your opinion to a corporation. Suppose the other person made lots of suggestions but ignored all the facts you had examined, what would you say?"

"It is difficult to handle complicated problems when you have a lot of experience and information. Impossible when you don't have either. I'd quietly suggest that the uninvited guest make no further suggestions until they were requested."

"Why not say the same to Jill?"

I do not plan what I am going to say to patients, and I do not know what sort of relationships we will develop. Toby and I were relatively close in age. We were outgoing, energetic professionals, with high standards and an intense concern with our careers. We loved life; family and friends were important to us both. I thought our shared interests would help us find common ground on which to build a relationship. But Toby rarely mentioned his work, his projects, or his family to me.

Despite his keen intelligence, his experience in solving problems, his confident use of logic, he had no interest in becoming my colleague in the management of his cancer. Although I gave him many opportunities to participate in the decision-making process, he wanted only to be my patient, to follow my advice, to live by my words.

The relationship between Toby and me was unique to us because we made it that way. In response to his cues, I felt myself reacting like a parent or a clergyman with him. He warmed to my efforts at being a gentle adviser, a strong supporter, a nurturer. He seemed to panic when I laid too much responsibility on his shoulders. When I revealed the vast ignorance that permeates the field of medicine, it frightened him. When I asked his advice about my plans to treat him, he looked perplexed.

"How am I supposed to know?" he asked. "You're the doctor!"

Toby was not the first mature, intelligent, informed, responsible individual to make it clear he wanted me to *be the doctor.* Medical decisions frightened him. Because he entrusted me with his life, because he believed his fate was in my hands, he could not tolerate the intimacy of a friendly relationship among equals. I was an authority, not a pal.

A judge recently told me, "Once a year I am assigned to the hospital to officiate in cases where an unresolved ethical issue has been referred to the courts for settlement. I gather information, select counsel to represent each party, listen to the arguments, and decide the issues. I follow an orderly procedure, including an appeal if necessary. But I *hate* making life-or-death decisions. The burden of responsibility disturbs my sleep. I agonize and grieve. Recently I made a decision I feel confident was correct. A woman who was nine months pregnant refused a Caesarean section. Without it, doctors feared both the woman and her baby would die. I listened carefully to both sides, but the choice was clear. I sided with the doctors. After the Caesarean section, both mother and baby lived. They are still thriving, but the mother hates me. I don't want to make any more decisions like that. My specialty is criminal law, not medicine!"

Medical decision making is not for everyone, even when the procedure is orderly and informed, the issues clear-cut, and consensus easy to obtain. As in soldiering, the participants fare better when they are mentally prepared.

Beatrice arrived in the emergency room and abruptly became my patient after a harrowing six-month experience with a series of physicians. It began with a routine physical examination.

"You should have a mammogram," her gynecologist told her.

"But I don't have any lumps," Beatrice replied.

"All the more reason to have a mammogram," the gynecologist said. "Nearly half of the breast cancers we find are in women who could feel no lumps. The cancers are the size of a pencil eraser, too small even for experienced physicians to feel, but lethal if not diagnosed early. We're saving many lives with mammograms. Be sure to get one soon!"

Dutifully, Beatrice obeyed her doctor. She was a meticulous accountant. She had a mammogram, although she did not have a family history of breast cancer and she felt well. To her shock and dismay, the mammogram showed a small cancer. Her gynecologist recommended a surgeon who specialized in breast diseases.

"Does this mean I am going to die?" she asked the surgeon.

The surgeon smiled at her ignorance.

"Highly curable," he said.

"But I thought cancer was always fatal," Beatrice said. The surgeon seemed aloof, unconcerned with her worries. She wondered if he were hiding the truth in order to spare her feelings. He seemed more inclined to deal with facts. Besides, he was a stranger. She did not feel comfortable talking about her feelings with strangers.

"The cancer you have is rarely fatal. In fact," the surgeon continued, "you have a choice of treatments. You can have a mastectomy or a lumpectomy followed by radiation therapy. It's up to you!"

"My God!" Beatrice thought. "Up to me? Cancer is a fatal illness. Radiation can cause cancer. I'm not even certain what a mastectomy is like. How could I ever decide?"

But the surgeon did not ask if she wanted to decide for herself or whether she felt comfortable securing several opinions. He terminated the discussion by turning her over to his receptionist, who proceeded to make appointments with a radiation therapist and a medical oncologist. Within a week, Beatrice had heard opinions from three doctors. Unfortunately, she did not feel she understood any of them well.

About that time, Beatrice began to experience severe headaches.

At first, she did not relate them to the illness. She had suffered from occasional headaches in the past. But the headaches began to come every day, to dominate her life with a miserable, unrelenting pain that ran from her right eyebrow to the back of her skull. They were only partially relieved by aspirin. When she mentioned the headaches to her surgeon, he interrupted the conversation.

"See your doctor about the headaches," he said. "My territory is the breast. I don't do heads, unless you want me to cut it off for you."

He chuckled as he continued writing notes in her chart. He did not notice Beatrice had failed to smile.

"I guess I'll go with the lumpectomy and radiation therapy," Beatrice said. "That way I'll get to keep my breast."

"It's fine with me," the surgeon said.

The surgery and radiation went well, according to both the surgeon and the radiation therapist. Beatrice found both to be a major nuisance. She had missed weeks of work for the first time in her life. She was disturbed by the constant probing and questioning. The surgeon and the radiation therapist never spoke with one another. Instead they communicated by letters that took a week or two to travel. No one resolved the minor differences in the instructions they had given her. Besides, the headaches had grown more persistent.

For the first time, Beatrice began to notice the medical bills. A self-supporting divorcée, Beatrice had never been seriously ill. Except for childbirth, she had never been in a hospital. Now she had bills for thousands of dollars from the mammographer, the surgeon, the consultants, the hospital, the radiation therapist, the pharmacy, the diagnostic radiologists, and the laboratories. The total cost was greater than her annual take-home pay.

"And all for a lump which was smaller than a lima bean," she said.

When the radiation therapy was completed, she visited a medical oncologist. He told her to take tamoxifen, a medication that would help control the cancer. He also told her that her platelet count was high.

"What are platelets?" Beatrice asked, mildly alarmed.

"They are tiny structures in the blood, cell fragments that help the blood to clot. Normally, there are a few hundred thousand of them in every cubic millimeter of blood. You have about a million of them. It's probably not dangerous, but it could be."

"Does it have anything to do with the breast cancer or the radiation?" Beatrice asked.

"I don't think so," the oncologist said. But he did not sound as certain as Beatrice would have liked.

During the next two months, the platelet count continued to rise. The oncologist seemed unconcerned. She became suspicious and consulted another oncologist.

The second oncologist shared Beatrice's concern about the platelets. In the next few weeks, he did several studies on Beatrice. While he was collecting information, her headaches became intense. Because of the pain, she could no longer concentrate on numbers or solve problems. She took a leave of absence from work. In tears, she appeared in the oncologist's office.

He discontinued the tamoxifen.

"Perhaps it is causing your headaches," he said.

"But won't I die without it?"

"It's not going to make much of a difference in your case," he told her.

The headaches grew worse. Fearful that the high platelet count had caused her headaches, the oncologist administered a platelet-suppressive medication. When the initial dose failed to have an effect, he increased it. Her platelet count remained unchanged, and so he admitted her to the hospital. By then, she was screaming because of the pain in her head and could not communicate clearly.

She was seen by several specialists and ultimately discharged with no clear diagnosis. By the time of discharge, her platelet count was normal, her white blood cells were dangerously low, and her headaches continued to be severe. Within a week of discharge, she arrived in the emergency room with a fever of 102°, seeking another opinion. Thus, at eleven o'clock one Friday night, our relationship began.

I had difficulty piecing the information together. Beatrice had consulted excellent physicians, each of whom had tried to give her clear explanations and assist her in making sensible decisions. Nevertheless, a year later, she still had dozens of unanswered questions about every element of her illness, questions that poured out amidst a flood of tears.

I spent two hours with her, answering each question. Gradually, the tears gave way to smiles of confidence.

"You're the first doctor who has explained things so I could understand," she said.

During her brief hospital stay, Beatrice's white blood count returned to normal, her fever disappeared, and her headache began to subside. After discharge, I arranged to see Beatrice in my office. By then, I had obtained reports from each of her doctors and held telephone conversations with them. I reviewed the reports and defined each problem. Although the physicians had attempted to sound professionally detached, I could detect a note of disapproval in their descriptions of Beatrice. She had fired two oncologists.

Over the next year, Beatrice's headaches gradually improved. She tried to return to work two or three times but was unable to withstand the pressure of full-time work until nearly six months after her surgery. By then, I had tried several analgesics, muscle relaxants, antidepressants, support groups, and psychotherapy. None of my suggestions had helped.

When Beatrice returned to my office, she told me her view of the illness.

"I couldn't stand the confusion, the contradictory medical advice, the misdiagnoses. You took the time to explain what was wrong with me. I had three problems, not one. The high platelet count was unrelated to the breast cancer. Depression about my medical problems caused my headaches. It would have helped if my doctors had talked with each other. Instead, I felt as if I had to give them information I did not understand myself. I was afraid

I would make a mistake. My fear worsened my depression and destroyed my trust in physicians. Without a sense of trust, I could not recover. It took months for me to be myself again."

Added to the challenge of forming relationships with my patients is the complex task of dealing with their companions. A colleague once told me to leave the companions in the waiting room. "If you're not careful, you will have to contend with a lot of extra anxiety and anger."

I ignored his advice. Bonds between people are an important source of strength in adverse times. My patients' companions could be more help if they had access to me. Listening to them was more than a kind gesture, it was a form of therapy.

Edgar and Mary always came to my office together. Mary had survived three threats to her life: bladder cancer, breast cancer, and hypertension. Edgar had shared every one of Mary's illnesses with her although he was unwell himself. Edgar had nerve deafness, macular degeneration, heart disease, and arthritis. He strained to hear our conversations. With the help of a magnifying lens, he could read the literature I gave him, but it took him hours. He wheezed as he trudged into my office, lurching despite the support of his cane. But he never let Mary come alone.

Mary developed bladder cancer long before I met her. It posed little threat at first. A superficial growth, the bladder cancer vanished after a urologist dosed her bladder with chemotherapy. The urologist was satisfied with the treatment and continued it for seven years. In his enthusiasm for controlling her bladder cancer, he failed to notice that the chemotherapy had caused incurable bone-marrow damage.

Mary became weak and short of breath. She consulted her internist. He discovered she had a severe anemia. He ordered an immediate blood transfusion, the first of more than one hundred units of blood that Mary was to receive in the next three years. Shortly after he discovered the anemia, the internist sent Mary to me.

At first sight, Mary and Edgar seemed like opposites. Mary, a quiet, earnest woman, had earthy, pointed questions about her problems. She liked practicality; although she often mentioned newspaper articles, she did not read medical journals. She accepted my answers with a trustful nod. Edgar talked incessantly, like a junior colleague anxious for acknowledgement. He never arrived without a string of questions about his wife's problems. He brought articles he had gleaned from various sources, some relevant, most not. He brought me literature searches from the National Library of Medicine and the Physician Data Query (PDQ). He provided me with a steady background of health-related material about people he knew. He gave evidence of being a frustrated physician, a man whose lack of a medical degree did not keep him from bursting with interest about medical science.

Mary wanted to return to normalcy. She would ignore her symptoms in order to weed her garden, cook meals, and see the ballet. She never doubted she would die from bone-marrow failure. She was content to delay death as long as possible.

Edgar longed for cure. Obsessed with what he believed was the life-saving potential of modern medicine, he combed the literature for an avenue of escape from Mary's fatal illness. No visit seemed to satisfy him without at least one suggestion of an alternative treatment not yet explored. He never failed to apologize for his intrusions into "my" specialty. He was discreet with his suggestions, informed as to the sources, armed with references if I wanted them.

Edgar laughed with ease, loved jokes and puns, and ridiculed himself with a deft tongue. Mary masked her emotions behind a dour face. Only rarely did she indulge herself in a grunt or a tight-lipped grin. She came to my office out of necessity. Her face was stern, and she greeted medical interventions such as blood transfusions with irritation. Although she usually tolerated Edgar's exuberant suggestions, on occasion she would silence him with annoyance.

Our relationship was strained at first. I did not know whether to appease Mary with practical advice or humor Edgar with dialogues about his hopeful speculations. With time, I discovered their flair for compromise. Despite their differences, they accepted each other's foibles. By participating in their relationship, I found it possible to appease Mary *and* humor Edgar.

Together, we probed the major issues regarding Mary's illnesses. We talked about how they happened and whether they could have been prevented. We wondered together how to go forward, how to manage each problem as it arose. We asked not only *what* we could do but *whether* we should do it. The discussions were sometimes heavy, full of pain for all of us, but more easily manageable because we were a cohesive unit.

Mary and Edgar had no children. Mary had family in Baltimore, but she rarely spoke with them. Edgar's family had been small, and none of his relatives still lived.

"Mary's all I've got," he told me.

I began to view Mary's illnesses as tragic beyond their consequences for her. Edgar's survivorship loomed on the horizon, his loneliness enhanced by his poor eyesight and impaired hearing. The bone marrow failure had more than one victim.

But Mary and Edgar, despite the load of illness, never appeared depressed. The awareness of the gravity of her illness challenged Mary to be optimistic and to outlive her prognosis.

"I may not last forever, but I'm going to last as long as I can. It's like W. C. Fields said about being dead and buried, Doctor, 'On the whole, I'd rather be in Philadelphia.' "

Edgar chortled, I laughed behind my hand, and Mary even cracked a smile. I discovered the couple's secret. They had a passion for old comic films, for W. C. Fields and Mae West, for Laurel and Hardy, for Charlie Chaplin and the Marx brothers. Together they could recite the lines by heart, replay the scenes, and laugh as heartily at the jokes as if they were new. On occasion they gave me tapes of the old shows as loving gifts.

When her final days arrived, Mary and Edgar looked upon each other with an affection which had grown during years of well-requited love. Each wished to spare the other the misery of the final days of her illness. Edgar sought to protect Mary from pain.

Mary wanted to avoid "appearing" ill, to conceal the degree to which the leukemia had ravaged her body. I perceived her caring heart thinly hidden behind a screen that might have been mistaken for vanity. She was obsessed with cleanliness and makeup, with groomed hair and fresh nightgowns. She wanted Edgar's memories to be sweet ones. On a rare occasion when they were apart, I spoke with Mary in her hospital room. With the only tears I ever saw her shed, she told me her biggest fear was that she could not protect Edgar from the pain of losing her. On his part Edgar, who cried easily, worried that Mary had never notified her family of her illness. She insisted it would do no one any good to worry about her. As time ran out, he convinced her it would be a great offense to her family if she kept the illness secret from them.

Mercifully, Mary died while she slept. The nurse found her while making rounds. She never experienced the agonies we had feared. I was on hand when Edgar arrived in the hospital. His eyes were dry.

"We did all we could, Doctor," he said. "Thank goodness she didn't suffer."

I hugged him hard and long and without embarrassment, although we were in the main corridor of the hospital. I, too, had lost a dear friend.

A year later, Edgar returned to our office for a visit. Clutched under his arm was a small package.

"Mary and I talked a lot about you, Doctor," Edgar told me. "We both agreed she had three good years that she would not have had without your efforts."

"You're looking well," I said.

"I manage," he replied. "I've discovered I had more friends in the community than I ever knew about. I rarely eat alone."

Edgar greeted everyone in our office, especially the nurses who had supported Mary through her years of illness. He was full of medical information for me. He had a catalog of stories about people with cancer, people he had met in the hospital while visiting Mary. Before he left, he handed me the package. While he watched, I unwrapped the videotape.

"I hope you like *You Can't Cheat an Honest Man*," he said. "It was always Mary's favorite."

Personal relationships have healing powers of their own, even when medications fail.

Maude, an eighty-year-old retired school teacher from rural Mississippi, developed cancer of the duodenum. The cancer grew until it blocked her intestine. After her surgeon had bypassed the blockage, he sent Maude to me for chemotherapy. I felt somewhat tentative about it. I knew I could not cure Maude's cancer. I could not even extend her life. I told her as much. But she felt she wanted to try chemotherapy even if the chance it would help her was slim.

"Slim's better'n nothin'," Maude said.

"In any case, it usually does not have side effects," I said. "The regimen I have in mind will not make you feel worse."

When I began her treatment, I had no means of measuring Maude's response. The cancer was located deep within her mammoth belly, beyond the reach of my probing fingers. Neither blood tests nor CAT scans gave any sign of cancer.

As we became acquainted, however, I discovered Maude's clinical response could easily be measured. I simply counted the number and variety of vegetables she produced in her garden. A Depression-era widow, the meager salary which Maude earned teaching school had barely sufficed to buy clothes. To survive, she had been forced to scratch for food on a tiny farm. She had raised vegetables with the fervor of a revivalist at a tent meeting. Although the years of necessity had long since passed, her commitment to her garden had not ebbed.

"This here tomato is a special variety. You can't get the seeds in any of the local stores. I have to send clear down to a supplier in Jackson for it. But I'll tell you, sure as the good Lord made little green apples, it's the best tomato you'll find to come ripe during Indian summer. The trouble with most tomatoes is they all come a-croppin' in August. Nothin' to do with 'em but can 'em. You can only eat so many tomatoes before you've had your fill of 'em. But a good tomato for late September is a treat."

"How does your abdomen feel today, Maude?" I asked.

"It's been giving me fits, 'specially after I been out to the garden weedin' and tyin' up tomatoes for two hours in that hot September sun."

"I tell her to stop," said her daughter. "But she won't listen to me."

I listened to the stories Maude loved to tell, not just about vegetables but about her life in Mississippi, her relationship with her daughter, the details living with cancer brought to mind. Just as she had learned to survive hardship in the past by concentrating on the tasks in front of her, she used housework, her garden, and her daughter's needs to divert her attention from the malignant growth inside her body, a growth we both knew could not be made to disappear.

As time passed, I recognized I had been wrong about treating Maude. My chemotherapy may not have helped her, but her frequent visits to my office did. I came to appreciate that my attention to her stories, my interest in her life, had helped give her the strength to endure her physical hardships. Knowing that a physician was interested in her had made it possible for her to function almost as well as she had before the cancer struck.

During the second winter after Maude first visited me, her energy began to flag. Together we made a decision to halt treatment "for a while."

"I need to take some weight off of these weary bones," she said.

One morning when I arrived in the office, I found two jars of tomatoes with a note.

> Thanks to you, Doctor, the crops are in. I want you to know how grateful I am for everything you've done.

I prepare for new encounters with the intensity of a concert soloist in rehearsal. Unless I perform at my best, the audience will be disappointed. I concentrate my thoughts, read, and review. Not until the interview is completed do I discover whether I have succeeded. Then either gentle applause or thundering silence announces the results of my efforts.

My audiences are families, clustered in my office. My performances, professional analyses of their illnesses and recommendations for treatment. I want my audiences to know the strength of my commitment to them, the world of science, and the healing art. I want each relationship I form to be ideal, but I know I cannot expect every one of them to succeed.

On a busy day, I may see three or four new patients, strangers to me, unknown except for their pathology reports and their X-ray films, their laboratory data and their healing scars. The surgeons have gotten to them before I ever see them. I miss the panic of the new diagnosis, the lump in the breast, the blood in the stool, the transition from healthiness to wondering whether it is foolish to buy a week's worth of groceries. Many of my patients first come to me after their surgery, and they want to know what to do next.

Some make do with a single visit if no other treatment is needed, but most see me more often. I examine them, order tests, initiate treatment, evaluate progress. The majority will see me more than half a dozen times a year. Some, in fact, will come several times a month.

One day I was asked to see two women in their forties, newly diagnosed with breast cancer. One was a divorcée, the other the wife of a friend of mine. I did not know either of them.

Pressed by my office schedule, I hurried to the hospital room where Shirley, the divorcée, was waiting with her friend Carole.

"Carole is the chairperson of my support group!" Shirley said.

Quickly I reviewed the clinical information with her. I wanted her to be clear about the facts I would use to formulate a plan.

She listened intently without a trace of distress. We mentioned the emotional strain more than once, but her emotions appeared to be under control. She told me her friends had helped her cope with the shock of learning she had cancer. Besides, her aunt and her grandmother had died from breast cancer. She was no stranger to the disease.

"A single lymph node in your armpit had cancer cells," I said. I discussed risks, used numbers to clarify relationships. I hid nothing.

"You are responsible for yourself," I said. "Even if it is painful, you must be in control of the facts."

Her work was important to her. She served as dean in a local college. In her work, she confronted malignant problems, too. Frustrated parents held her at bay while they vented their anger at the college and their recalcitrant children. They expected her to respond, to show concern, to care. To meet those expectations, she needed energy and enthusiasm. I promised to do my best to keep her pert and snappy.

Her physical appearance had more than narcissistic value for her. Her job required her to spend many hours before audiences of parents and prospective students. As dean, she represented the college in other schools where her confident smile and crisp good looks helped her to recruit applicants.

"Can I do it with a wig?" she asked, half laughing.

"Are you all right?" Carole asked. Shirley nodded, but I could see tears forming in the corner of her eye.

"Stay beautiful," I said. "It's important. Besides, it will keep people from giving you those yucky looks of pity when you reenter their world. Maybe you'll miss hearing a few of those sad stories you didn't ask to be told."

I told her about women who had coped well with breast cancer while they fought to survive. Their gutsy gestures helped them manage to avoid humiliation when people offered them unwanted sympathy rather than respect. After we laughed heartily together, I departed.

I was a few minutes late for a conference at the hospital. Indeed,

I might have skipped the conference, but it was a memorial lecture for a friend, a physician who had died from cancer a year earlier.

As I sat in the darkened room, thoughts of my dead colleague crowded out the words of the lecturer. He had been young and determined, compassionate yet feisty. I do not know what he told others about his cancer, but often, when he met me in the hall, he regaled me with horror stories, disparaging of my specialty.

"You can't imagine what it's like," he said. "Most of you have no idea what you are doing to people. For the kind of cancer I have, chemotherapy is worthless, but I took it anyway. I figured I had nothing to lose. But the people who gave it to me made mistakes. I felt I had to watch them constantly."

His anger sparked guilty feelings even though he was not my patient, even though his doctors had done their best for him. He had been denied nothing. He had enjoyed three years of productive life before the cancer suddenly grew back. Yet both of us were disappointed because of the impotence of medicine in the face of his disease.

As I listened to the lecture in his honor, the memory of his death renewed my sense of loss at his passing. I remembered conversations with his patients, who described him as unusually compassionate. A rare physician with a rare cancer.

After the lecture, I hurried back to my office. Because I was late, I apologized for keeping Matthew and Lynne waiting. I explained where I had been. Matthew, who was also a physician, had also been a close friend of the doctor whose memorial lecture I had just attended, yet neither of us mentioned the event. Rather, our thoughts were focused on a current concern. Matthew's wife, Lynne, had just been discharged from the hospital after a mastectomy for breast cancer.

Like Shirley, Lynne craved information. She looked detached. Her emotions were hidden behind a cool exterior. Although Matthew had hinted in the hallways of the hospital about the tension she expressed at home, he said nothing about his feelings, either.

Her eyes were dry, her brow unwrinkled. She had done her homework—not only read the books but understood them. Her questions were cogent, her grasp of clinical information sound.

At her side, but slightly to her rear, Matthew listened in silence while we talked. Matthew and I shared a philosophy about medicine. Both of us were aware that the difficulty of our work paled in comparison to the struggles of our patients. We knew our patients were forced to cope with the uncertainty of their survival, the misery of having tests and taking medication, and the humiliation of losing independence, stature, and power. We both believed in lightening those burdens by educating our patients.

Lynne was in my office because Matthew had given her my name. Perhaps he had told her he respected me as a physician. I shuddered at the thought that he might have painted an overly enthusiastic view of me as meticulous, thoughtful, and willing to communicate. Fortunately, he made it clear that the choice of oncologists was hers to make. This encounter was a competitive audition.

I wanted to be at my best, not only because my performance was being observed by a colleague but because I wanted to help them. Deep inside, I felt my body balking. Indeed, for days before the event, I had felt an unusual tension. Although I enjoy working with patients and have cared for hundreds of women with breast cancer, I knew I was ambivalent about treating Lynne.

I did not even realize I felt ambivalent until we were seated in my office. Yet watching her, I could not avoid thinking about my own wife. Lynne's pert disposition, her lovely clothes, her gentle voice, her uncompromising intelligence, her professional achievements, her love of dance, and her dignified bearing reminded me of my wife. With her physician-husband seated beside her, it was almost impossible to avoid recalling a trip my wife and I had made to another doctor's office. Although my wife's nodule had not been a cancer, the clear memory of the episode awakened within me the tension I had felt, if only momentarily. Coupled with my freshly awakened grief for my dead colleague, I had lost my ability to concentrate on Lynne's needs and forget about my own.

I had not formed a relationship with Lynne. Because I knew Matthew as a colleague, I had not taken the time to become acquainted with her. Instead, I had talked *about* cancer with her, as if lecturing to a group of colleagues.

Skillfully, or so I thought at the time, I avoided any mention of my own concerns. Seeking to shield the couple from my ambivalence, I "communicated" about cancer, belaboring the details of the diagnosis, the prognosis, and the treatment plan. For more than forty minutes I rambled on, unable to alter my approach in response to Lynn's fixed expression and Matthew's grimaces. Too late, I became aware that mine was the only voice. I had violated a rule I hold dear: I had delivered a lecture instead of holding a conference. Desperately, I tried to extricate myself.

"Is there anything you'd like to know?" I asked Lynne. "I haven't given you much of a chance to talk." In fact, I hadn't given her any chance to talk. Anxiety, not wisdom, had unsurped the governance of my tongue.

"Keep going," she said. "You're on a roll."

"Is it all right?" I asked.

"I'm fine," she said.

I continued, covering yardage about causes and future prospects, treatment strategies, statistics. I was, if nothing else, both erudite and voluble. But I was never honest about my feeling: I was frightened because I was afraid to "fail." If nothing I did helped Lynne, I would be forced to watch her perish. No likelihood of cure could rid my mind of the image of some dire, untoward event that would steal the bloom from her cheek, erase her hair, destroy her ability to dance, reduce to helplessness this woman whose vivacity and beauty made even the possibility of cancer seem an offense to nature. Instead of attending to my patient, my mind was on my own wife, the woman who looks to me with cheerful trust, and I feared lest my best offerings be as worthless to her as those of others had been to my dead colleague.

In the end, we parted on a friendly note, sincere but reserved. I had made my recommendation, but I did not expect her to return. In the hallway, as we shook hands, I felt disappointed with myself.

A week later I received a handwritten note from Matthew. Lynne had found another doctor who proposed the same treatment

I had suggested. Perhaps, he speculated, the other oncologist had made Lynn more comfortable because he had asked Matthew to sit in the waiting room while he spoke to her.

I am not always at my best. Such experiences help to make me aware of my vulnerability to failure. I have faced life-threatening decisions with courage, calming others rather than yielding to my own fear. But on that day, when I was with Lynne and Matthew, discussing a cancer with a high prospect of cure, I was overcome by my awe of the fragile tendrils with which we cling to life.

I relish meeting new people, even if they have cancer. I want to do my best for them. Yet even with practice, my task is harder than that of a virtuoso performing Bach's cello suites. My "critics" analyze my every gesture, chance remark, and expression. But I am not a trained performer. I am living through the experience with them.

In developing relationships with people who came to me as patients, I met my match in Lou. He measured every inch of me, probed in depth about my family, my professional relationships, my aspirations. He discussed my children, analyzed my interest in the hospital's cancer program, and took vicarious pleasure when I went sailing and skiing. In fact, Lou was at his best when he was giving advice to me. He told me to use restraint as a parent, to love my children even when I was offended by their behavior. He made suggestions about the cancer program at the hospital. When he discovered I was planning to attend a medical meeting in Bermuda, he gave me detailed information about the island.

But his most abiding concern was that I stick with the struggle to help people live with cancer. He refused to allow his cancer cells to change his personality or dampen his enthusiasm for life.

At times, I found Lou long-winded. His verbosity tended to increase when his medical condition worsened. He used conversation to hold me in his presence as if he were afraid each meeting would be our last. Often I found I had to cut him off by promising I would return.

But there was a darker side to our relationship. For although Lou insisted upon being realistic, his illness was a fatal one. His sixty-year-old body had but months to live, a traitor to his intact mind. He accepted the fact of his death, but he refused to accept the process of dying. Each time his body tried to die, his mind fought with unusual vigor to delay the end, amazing onlookers with his tenacity for life. After one such miraculous survival, he wrote me a letter which he wanted to share with other people who had a fatal cancer. The text follows:

TO ALL PATIENTS WHO HAVE A TERMINAL ILLNESS

"I have cancer."

These three words are the second most important phrase that a victim of cancer can bring himself to say. Surely "I love you!" is much more important than that. When I finally forced myself to say "I have cancer," my whole life changed.

Although I was terrified when my doctor diagnosed my lymphoma, I soon realized that it was a blessing in disguise. For over a year I had been suffering from symptoms my doctor did not understand. I had anemia, a kind of swelling called edema, mysterious fevers, and constant fatigue. To my surprise, lymphoma explained everything. After the treatment was started, my ailments improved. I felt myself again.

More important than the treatment was the fact that my doctor always told me and my family everything there was to know about the lymphoma. He explained the treatment choices, including experimental therapies. Whenever I had a question, it was answered. Chemotherapy has been vital to keeping me alive and making me feel well. I recognize that I will probably never be cured, but each new day sparkles like a jewel on black velvet. When I first found out about the lymphoma, I had no grandchild. Since then, I have witnessed the birth of my granddaughter and watched her grow up to be a beautiful six-and-a-half-year-old. I have treasured every day of her precious life.

Even though there is no cure, I am content to control my disease and live with chemotherapy, hospital stays, and home confinement during my low-white-count days. It may not be a perfect life, but it's a whole lot better than the alternative!

Whenever one form of chemotherapy stops working for me, I have willingly agreed to go on to the next, after my doctor has explained the risks. I want to live as long as possible, and I am willing to take risks to live. But I have made up my mind about life support. I will never allow any physician to keep me alive on machines. I don't mind fighting to live, but when the fight has gone out of me, I want to go out with it.

"I have cancer" is enough for me to live with. I never say "I have death!" That's quite a different thing.

Remember to tell people who are afraid to say "I have cancer" to add "But it can be treated. Don't let it kill you without trying to help yourself!"

With the reader's indulgence, I would like to add a letter of my own.

Dear Lou,

Because of your letter, our many conversations, your thoughtful advice to me about how I should raise my children, manage my office, plan my vacations, and avoid being a workaholic, I will never forget you.

Like you, I wish we could have continued for many more years, while your granddaughter grew to adulthood and you battled, not just your cancer, but your diabetes, heart failure, increasing blindness, and kidney failure. I wish we could have gone from remedy to remedy, eking out a few more months of time. You came back once or twice when we thought your tired body had had enough. Neither of us could cheerfully accept the forces of nature that forbade you to continue.

But although we knew our relationship could not long endure, we did not care less for each other. We never blamed each other for something neither of us could prevent. Rather we cherished the hours we had together because we knew, as too few humans do, the preciousness of time.

5
ANXIETY

The only thing we have to fear is fear itself.
—Franklin Delano Roosevelt*

A FEELING of panic is decidedly unpleasant. It makes our heads ache, our blood pressure rise, our hearts race, our stomachs churn, our bowels and bladders evacuate. It makes us pant, sweat, grimace, tremble, and cry. When we are anxious, we can neither concentrate nor remember. We are disorganized, inattentive, and inaccurate. At the extreme, we may digress into nonsense, appear to listen but hear nothing, become mute or babble incessantly. Anxiety renders us irrational to the point that we may injure people who are attempting to help us.

The contagion of anxiety is well known. We spread it quickly to our family members and friends. We give it to doctors and nurses who care for us, and they reinfect us. Gripped by anxiety, groups of us have trampled each other to death.

*First Inaugural Address (March 4, 1933).

Before we met, I knew that Toby had developed acute anxiety. While I listened to Dr. Starch outside his room, I could sense anxiety from the rigidity of Toby's body, his worried face, and the dancing waves on the cardiac monitor.

The story of the events helped underscore the root of his anxiety. From Dr. Starch, I learned that Toby's cancer had been a surprise. For months doctors and patient had been satisfied that inflammation was responsible for his symptoms. They believed they had eliminated the possibility of cancer with appropriate tests. Toby's sudden awareness of the fallibility of medical technology added to the shock of learning he was going to die from cancer. His doctors were disturbed as well. For although physicians confront the fallibility of medical technology on a daily basis, it never ceases to create anxiety, particularly when a life is at stake.

Dr. Starch recovered his equilibrium. He derived confidence from using the same tests on other patients with more success. Although Toby's misfortune disturbed him, Dr. Starch did not forsake the technology that usually worked, even if it occasionally failed.

Toby's shock and disappointment lingered, however, because he had lost confidence in medicine, because he did not want to lose control of his life, because death did not fit into his plans. Cancer had denied him an expectation of future life, the delayed diagnosis had destroyed his confidence in physicians. Because lung cancer had been his only serious illness as an adult, he had no memory of past successes with medical care to buoy his confidence. Although he had heard of the miracles of modern medicine, happy stories about others did little to allay his fears. He felt like an exception to every rule.

To find clues which might help him to succeed in untying the anxious knots in Toby's head, I needed to know more about him. From Ginny I learned details about Toby's managerial role at work. He was an assertive leader, a clear thinker, a respected consultant.

He was ambitious and courageous. He enjoyed challenges. He set high goals and forced himself to achieve them.

"The man you see in the hospital is very different from the man I have known so many years," she said.

I could understand her concern about the changes in Toby. He looked frightened. His speech was jumpy, scattered, hard to comprehend. He could not set goals. His thoughts were disorganized, even inappropriate. Indeed, I often felt that he wanted me to tell him not to worry, to assure him that I would find a cure, to promise him that he could jog again. He rarely asked for facts. Rather, with a gesture or a glance, he would direct me to comfort him. He used me as a shield against the lung cancer he was afraid to discuss. Led more by compassion than the discipline of my profession, I yielded to his wishes. Although I felt deprived of the frankness that open discussion would have given us, the terror in his mournful eyes beseeched me to delay it.

I never lied to Toby. I never avoided an opportunity to talk. We talked often and well. But our conversations were accompanied by artful diplomacy.

"How long am I going to be able to function?" Toby would ask.

"What do you mean by that?" I would return, being careful not to tell him more than he wanted to know.

"Do you think I am going to suffer?"

"What kind of suffering did you have in mind?"

"Will I be in pain?"

"I have no way of knowing, but if pain develops, we have effective medications, and I will not hesitate to use them."

Instead of pushing me for details, he tended to digress, to tell me about himself, to forget that he had questions to ask. In time we became better acquainted, he learned my language, responded to me as a caring person rather than as a harbinger of the inky blackness that lay ahead.

Our conversations ranged over many topics, IBM and Operation Desert Storm, our families and people we admired. We talked about his symptoms. By working on his current problems, Toby adapted to his cancer. Each time we met, I listened for signals that he felt more comfortable talking with me. As each day passed, I gently reminded him that the cancer was still our major issue, one we would be forced to discuss. I never let my fear of his emotions prevent me from making eye contact with him. I maintained a steady voice, touched his hand, and responded to his need for comfort. I pretended I was certain his anxiety would quickly fade.

"Am I going to die?" he asked on the third day.

In the seconds that followed, a dozen thoughts rushed through my mind. Messages beyond words seemed to flow between the two of us. He wanted a simple answer to his question. One word would have sufficed. Yet I felt a tug within me, a tug that made me refine the answer I knew he would remember forever. It was not my reply, but my choice of words that he would carry in his heart. I wanted to share the burden of his poor prognosis without pronouncing a death sentence upon him. I wanted my words to be part of his knowledge, not a penalty for having inquired about a subject best left to God.

"You know as well as I do that lung cancer is usually fatal," I said softly. He nodded like a colleague.

Time did not permit me to quell Toby's anxiety. I urged the Thompsons to work with a psychiatric nurse, who was able to help them through the crisis. With her guidance, Toby and his family were able to acknowledge his approaching death. He spoke frankly about the need to settle his affairs. In a calm voice Toby gave counsel to his wife and children. The nurse felt certain Toby had accepted the fact that he would die from cancer.

Yet although he could speak about his death in the presence of his family, he continued to look terrified when I talked about it. It was as if my words and my voice had a special meaning for him. I remarked to the psychiatric nurse about the awesome effect I had on Toby.

"If it's the same message, what does it matter who says it?" I asked.

"I'm a Catholic," she said. "I know that telling a friend about something I've done wrong feels very different from going to confession."

Two weeks after discharge from the hospital, Toby came to my office to discuss plans for chemotherapy. I planned to explain the details of his treatment to him. I chose highly toxic therapy with the knowledge that less potent medications would be of little help. His chances remained slim even with the more toxic combination. Because it was strange to him, I expected Toby to have many questions about the medications and their side effects.

From the moment he arrived, I sensed his anxiety. His voice cracked as he spoke, and his eyes darted around the room. He seemed unable to wait for answers to his insistent questions before asking others. To my surprise the chemotherapy was of relatively little concern to him.

"What about this tube, Doctor? Can't it come out?"

In my enthusiasm for starting treatment, I had nearly forgotten the small tube we had left in his chest.

"But Toby, we left it there for your comfort. We wanted to prevent the pleural fluid from collecting. If the fluid reaccumulates, it will make you short of breath."

"There's no fluid coming out any more, Doctor. Can't it be removed?"

My efforts to distract him from the tube were fruitless. Because I had other patients to see, I had limited time to allow him to digress. I wanted to concentrate on my own agenda. But Toby's demands were unrelenting.

I saw the tube as a minor distraction, a tiny addition to his physical burden. It was soft, flexible, and painless. It was invisible when he was dressed. I wanted him to ignore it.

But Toby loathed the tube, a constant reminder of his cancer. His mouth twisted in an angry grimace, as he growled about the miserable mess created by the tiny tube. The covering had been inadequate. It had been impossible to keep dry. His clothes were soiled by it. He hated the tube. He wanted it removed.

"The tube is worse than living with death," he told me.

Instinct told me to acquiesce rather than press for victory. Besides, if the mere presence of the tube annoyed Toby, it would be difficult for me to convince him he should keep it in for comfort.

I removed the tube.

Medicine is, at best, an uncertain art. Our behavior is even more unpredictable than the processes at work in our bodies. People whose lives are filled with anxiety may meet calamity with unexpected serenity. A woman I knew reacted to every new event in her life with terror. She wondered whether she might have caught AIDS by riding on the subway or passed cancer to her grandchildren because of germs she might have spread to them. Yet when her first grandchild died suddenly in its crib, she remained supremely calm, and when she developed cancer herself, her anxiety was replaced by tender concern for her husband.

In my efforts to become familiar with the families of my patients, I often identify the "reactor" in the group, a person who serves as the barometer of familial distress. While the rest of the family remains composed, flames and smoke hiss from the reactor's nostrils. Mary Lou and Jerry were such a pair.

"You'll have to talk to Jerry," Mary Lou said when I returned her call. "I just don't feel comfortable talking about it."

If Mary Lou was too upset to talk, I expected Jerry to scream into the telephone. Jerry had a hair-trigger temper, while Mary Lou was almost sugary sweet, docile in her acceptance of frightening news. At least they had behaved that way when Mary Lou was in the hospital. While she summoned Jerry to the telephone, thoughts of our previous encounters buzzed through my brain.

A year earlier, I had admitted Mary Lou to the hospital because she had a cough and chest pain. Although she did not smoke, I was concerned about the possibility of cancer. Her chest X-ray had been suspicious. I explained my plans to both of them. I waited while they asked questions. I arranged for Mary Lou to have a bronchoscopy. Mary Lou smiled sweetly throughout the discussion. Jerry said nothing.

The following morning, the transporter arrived to take Mary Lou for the procedure. She signed the consent form and nodded that she was ready to go.

"What the hell is happening?" Jerry roared in the hallway as Mary Lou slid onto the gurney. "That's *my* wife you're taking away. I demand to know where she's going!"

From my seat at the nursing station, I could hear the eruption. I finished writing in a chart and hurried over to talk to Jerry. By the time I reached him, Mary Lou had disappeared into the elevator, but his anger had not yet abated.

"She lies in bed suffering, and you do nothing to help her!" he screamed at me. I reminded him of the treatments I had prescribed, of the diagnostic tests, of the consultations I had obtained. He greeted each of my comments with scorn and distrust. I felt the blood rushing to my head and gut. Only my dignity and my commitment to helping people kept me from losing my temper.

By the time of his wife's discharge, Jerry had become friendlier. Although he never embraced the system and never seemed to understand clearly what I was doing for Mary Lou or why I was doing it, he was pleased to see her well.

I did not know what new problem Mary Lou had developed. But I expected Jerry to erupt in anger if the problem was too severe for Mary Lou to talk about.

"What happened, Jerry?" I asked, hiding my disbelief that his was the cooler of the two heads.

"The doctor found a cancer in her uterus," he said. To my surprise his voice was steady. "He's going to take it out next Wednesday. Mary Lou wanted you to know."

"Her gynecologist called me," I told him. "It's an early cancer, Jerry. I expect Mary Lou will do quite well from what her doctor told me. Surgery alone should be enough to cure her. If it isn't, we can talk about it later."

"I know, Doctor," Jerry said. "Her gynecologist explained everything to me. I'm not worried, but I wish you'd tell her how you feel. Ever since we left the doctor's office, she's been shaking like a leaf." He handed the receiver back to his wife.

Mary Lou's voice trembled. She was unable to talk. She could not bring herself to say the word *cancer*. Indeed, when I started to talk about the tumor, she begged me to stop. Rather than arouse her even further, I spoke briefly in a soothing tone.

"I am glad you are in good hands," I said. "I expect you will do beautifully."

Sometimes I am misled in my efforts to be gentle. I see people crying. I suspect that what I am saying is the cause. I do not want to distress them. Then, just as in the midst of surgery a careful surgeon must tie a severed vessel before proceeding with an operation, I must take stock of the situation before deciding whether to end the conversation.

Not long ago I ushered Bette and Ralph into my office for a discussion.

"I asked you to come today because I wanted to talk to you about your cancer," I said. Ralph remained stony-faced, but he did not look at me. Bette reached into her pocketbook for a tissue.

"Dr. Mills has told you that the biopsy confirmed the diagnosis of breast cancer," I continued. Ralph's face did not change. Bette's eyes suffused with tears.

"You will need further surgery," I said. Ralph remained impassive. Bette blew her nose loudly.

"This conversation seems to be upsetting you," I said. "Perhaps I should stop." Ralph said nothing.

"Please don't stop, Doctor," Bette said. "You're doing fine. I want to hear all of the facts. I can't help crying, but I still want to know. If I force myself not to cry, I won't be able to concentrate on what you have to say."

"By the way, Doctor," Ralph added, his face still frozen in stony coldness. "I'm more emotional than Bette is, I just don't know how to show it."

Anxiety can be adaptive. Fear of traffic helps prevent accidents. Fear of the law keeps us honest. Fear of public disapproval helps us to be more sociable.

Even fear of cancer can be helpful. Fear prompts people to submit to physical examinations, mammography, and other cancer screening tests, despite their discomfort and expense. Fear of cancer helps people conquer their addiction to cigarettes. Fear directs us to seek treatment early, to heed medical advice, to pay attention to details.

In our country, where self-restraint is deemed a virtue, emotions like anxiety are only tolerated in small doses. We want to believe strength of character will prevent us from "giving in" to anxiety. Few of us escape from the tendency to be prejudiced against "chickens." We honor soldiers who have "conquered" fear and heap scorn upon those who yielded to their anxiety. War veterans know the truth: what seems like courage is often a matter of luck. Heroism plays only a small part. Each of us has a breaking point.

Our emotions are not like a gas flame, which can be controlled by a knob. They are more like a forest fire, which spreads when the conditions are right. Few of us know the conditions that will unleash the fire of our own anxiety. Much less do we understand those conditions in other people.

"I once spent a night in a twin-engine plane," a federal agent told me. "I was surrounded by heavily armed revolutionaries chanting anti-American slogans. I knew they wanted to kill me, yet I was able to concentrate on writing a detailed report for the Agency. The possibility of imminent death didn't frighten me, Doctor. It was all in a day's work. But a rectal examination scares the hell out of me!"

"I feel ridiculous," Cindy told me as she fumbled for the box of tissues. "Before I got cancer, I never let anyone see how I felt about things. My boyfriend used to call me the Iceberg. I was so good at hiding my feelings that I often didn't know I had them. I'd see something frightening or infuriating or heart-wrenching, but I would let it pass by. Within minutes it would be almost forgotten. I certainly would never have cried in a doctor's office.

"It's been three years since I had my mastectomies. I never grieved for my breasts. With my family history, I almost expected to lose them. You men seem to think every woman is infatuated with her breasts. Let me set you straight. They didn't matter much to me. I'd rather be alive any day than walk around hoping some man would admire by boobs. As far as I'm concerned, they were a glorified lunch counter. I don't miss them a bit! It's just that . . . "

Her voice stopped abruptly. She reached for another tissue.

" . . . I feel a sense of panic whenever I am in a crowd or have a deadline I can't meet or discover my bank account has gotten low. I'm not just worried anymore. I'm petrified. I don't understand it."

Cindy had arrived in my office three years earlier, not long after she discovered her breast cancer. She had never been ill. She was slim and attractive. She had two teenaged daughters, but her husband, whom she referred to as her third child, had deserted her for a neighbor half his age.

"You're in great shape," I had told her when I finished my examination. "You've never had any serious illness; you don't smoke or drink; you don't take any medications. But you mentioned something about cancer in your family. Tell me about it."

"When I was about fourteen, my mother developed breast cancer. She was uneducated. She was terrified of doctors. She hid it from me as long as she could, but I caught a glimpse of it one Sunday. We were on the way to Mass, and I was helping her into her dress. I was frightened, but I knew I couldn't let my mother see how I felt. Her emotions were so delicate that I was afraid she would fall apart. So I acted strong. I put my arm around her and told her not to worry. Then I tried to convince her to go to a doctor, but she refused.

" 'God will take care of me,' she said. She glanced at the icons on the mantelpiece. Then she picked up the pastries she had baked for church. I knew the conversation was finished.

"By the time Mama went to a doctor, the cancer had spread around her chest from front to back. The surgeon just shook his head and didn't say anything for a while. Then he looked at me.

" 'How old are you, young lady?'

"I told him.

" 'Are you her only child?'

"I told him I was the only family Mama had.

" 'Then you will have to learn to give her injections of morphine,' he said.

"I had to nurse Mama until she died. Even with the morphine, the pain was terrible. She could not eat. She was only thirty-eight years old when she died. Her younger sister died of breast cancer a few years later."

Cindy had shown no trace of emotion as she recalled her mother's illness. I noted the family history in the chart and returned to Cindy's problem.

It had been a small growth with a high prospect of permanent cure. With careful study, we came to the conclusion that both breasts should be removed in order to minimize her risk of recurrent disease.

Our conversations about her illness had sounded entirely objective. Her emotional detachment made me shiver. If a man had come into my office waiting room looking for the Iceberg, no one would have doubted he meant Cindy.

She had undergone surgery without complaint. Within two weeks she returned to my office to begin adjuvant chemotherapy, a form of treatment designed to prevent the return of her cancer, although, to our great satisfaction, all of her test results gave promise that she might have been cured by surgery. Throughout the six-month course of chemotherapy, she never complained or cried.

"I'm an attorney," she had told me. "I've seen worse things happen to other people. I'll be all right."

The panic attacks had begun a year later. They were infrequent at first. She handled them by making a quick retreat to the ladies' room to "wash her face." When she doused herself with cold water, she usually regained emotional control within a few minutes.

Over the following months, however, the attacks became more frequent. She felt compressed by crowds. An evening's entertainment at the Kennedy Center would be destroyed in the foyer as she brushed elbows with other ticket holders. Her smile of anticipation would rapidly dissolve in tears.

"I would cry for no reason," she told me. "I was so humiliated that I quit attending performances even though I had season tickets to the ballet."

As she sat in my office, describing her problem, I thumbed through her chart looking for clues.

"I wonder," I asked her, "is it important that today is your thirty-eighth birthday?"

"You don't understand, Doctor," Cindy said. "I'm not going to get sentimental about my mother, not after all these years. I never yield to my emotions."

"Well, I do," I said. "I laugh at comedies. I cry at tragedies. I hate the villain and admire the hero. When I get sick, I get scared, too. Every time I get a bad headache, I wonder if I have a brain tumor or a hemorrhage. My feelings are even stronger when my wife or children are sick. My emotions tell me where I am. They give me a clue to the significance of what is happening to me. I think they help me adapt to change. Sometimes I can hide them, but I can't control them. And I'm not embarrassed to have them.

"Your panic attacks are a problem, not an embarrassment. They are an illness, not a sign of moral weakness."

A few months later, using a combination of psychotherapy and medication, Cindy's problem disappeared.

115

ANXIETY

If I had a sure remedy for anxiety, I would not have the leisure to write about it. My office would be crammed with high-paying customers willing to "give away the ranch" in exchange for relief from this distressing emotion. The formula that helped Toby conquer his anxiety could not be generalized. What worked well for Toby Thompson failed miserably for Paula Petrie.

"Please talk to Mrs. Petrie," Dr. Block had told me.

"What's the problem?"

"She has a breast cancer. I think she should have a mastectomy, but I gave her the options. See what you think. Look at the slides and the mammogram. I'll send you everything you need. And one more thing, Dan, try to talk some *sense* to her."

"I'll do my best."

The alarm in Dr. Block's voice was clear. He told me he had met Mrs. Petrie twice. She had brought her husband. Each time he had spent an hour delineating the options. He had drawn pictures, shown them journal articles, talked in terms of probabilities and expectancies, risks and benefits. Each time he had asked probing questions at the end of the session. Each time the Petries seemed to be confused.

I planned to give the Petries a one-hour appointment. I arranged with my receptionist to place the appointment at the end of the day. If I needed more time, I would be able to extend their visit without keeping other patients waiting.

The Petries arrived with a clutch of papers and radiology jackets dating back several years. Side by side, they sat in my conference room, not touching, scarcely looking at each other.

"What can I do for you?" I asked.

They both started to talk at once, caught themselves, fell silent again. Mrs. Petrie nodded to her husband.

"Perhaps you ought to tell him. You are the articulate one. I get all tongue-tied when it comes to medical information."

Mr. Petrie started to describe in exasperating detail the mechanics of making appointments and switching them, of the treatment they received in the parking lot and the waiting room, as if I could help them with the frustrations in their lives, which were as much beyond my control as theirs. Never once did he mention the words *breast* or *cancer* or *surgery* or *radiation therapy*.

I glanced through Mrs. Petrie's folder while he described with great irritation an impertinent receptionist who kept him on hold for five minutes, then cut him off and blamed the disconnection on his impatience.

Both of the Petries were tenured members of the faculty of a nearby university. She was an expert in Japanese art, and he was a professor of music. He performed off campus in a chamber group which was well known in the city. I had heard him play recently.

"I enjoyed the Beethoven concert you played two weeks ago," I said.

His mouth curled in a tight smile, and for a few seconds he seemed about to interrupt himself.

"I think we'd better stick to talking about Paula's cancer, don't you?" he said.

I nodded and listened while he continued his meticulous descriptions of incidentals that played no part in making a decision about his wife's cancer. He described the paintings on the wall of the surgeon's waiting room.

"I used the last piece of toilet paper in their bathroom," he said. "I think it should be stocked better than that. His fees are high enough!"

"Has he sent you a bill?" I asked.

"Not yet. But I know it will be a big one!"

I hoped to gain more information by encouraging Mrs. Petrie to talk about her problem.

"When did you first find the lump?" I asked her.

"That's just it," she said. "I never found a lump."

"Tell me about it," I asked.

"I went for a routine physical examination because I had not had one in fifteen years. I felt well. I was finished having babies. I didn't have any good reason for having an examination. It just seemed like a good idea. My mother had died of breast cancer when she was the same age I am now. She suffered terribly with it. It got into her bones and lungs. She had months of pain and starvation. I used to bathe her. When she was too weak to sit up, I fed her with a spoon. She had been a fiercely independent woman. Raised three children with no husband. My father was hit by a truck when my younger brother was not even two years old. We owed a lot to her. I never begrudged taking care of her, but all the same I learned to hate cancer. It's a dreadful disease. I'll never forget what she told me."

"What was that?"

"She had had a particularly bad day. She had cried because of the pain. She made me lean over so she could whisper in my ear.

" 'I pray every day that you will never get cancer,' she said. Those were her last words to me. The next day she died."

Abundant ironies hung in the air, although no one spoke about them. The pain of long-ago hidden grief, reawakened by a daughter's recapitulation of her mother's illness. The sudden challenge to her faith, the failure of her mother's prayers. Poignant reminders of the darker possibilities of life and the futility of passionate desire to prevent them.

She told me about her mammogram, which, to everyone's surprise, had shown a suspicious calcification, a tiny star-shaped spot that signaled a new growth, probably a cancerous one.

"Many of them cannot be felt with fingers," I told her.

"But I feel so well," she protested. "My mother looked terrible. She lost so much weight that her skin hung loose around her face. She had always been a beautiful woman, much more beautiful than I. The cancer stole her looks."

"You should feel well," I said. "Your cancer has been found at a stage much earlier than your mother's generation dared hope for. We use mammograms to find cancers when they are still too small to find with the fingers in the hopes that the growth is limited to the breast."

"I know that," she said and twisted in her chair.

"I'm sorry. I didn't mean to be pedantic."

After she had described the course of events which had led her to my office, I examined her and then the mammograms. I agreed with the surgeon. I thought the small calcified area should be removed. If the piece that was removed was surrounded with a clear margin of normal breast tissue, free of cancer cells, she might be treated with radiation therapy and spared a total mastectomy. In fact, I hoped surgery would suffice. On the contrary, if the cancer were more extensive, then a mastectomy would be required.

When I had finished considering the information, I proceeded to discuss the options, examining the risks and benefits of each and emphasizing the contingencies upon which the advice rested. They listened intently, interrupting for questions. I felt at ease with them and allowed the discussion to continue for more than an hour.

"Do you feel settled now?" I asked when I had finished.

"Not at all!" Mrs. Petrie said. The harshness of her voice echoed her visible annoyance. "I don't understand why you can't make up your minds. All I ask is clear advice, and all you do is say, 'If this, then that.' Can't you just tell me what to do?"

Anger suffused her face with a deep red glow. I thought of the Chinese saying, "Anger opens the mouth and closes the eyes." I turned to her husband in search of friendly support, but his face was turned to the wall. Suddenly he shrugged.

"We might as well leave, dear," he said, grabbing his hat and coat as he rose from his chair. "You know they never tell you anything."

"I hate anxious patients," Kenneth told me.

"I didn't ask you how you felt about the patient," I said, a little sharply. "I asked you to take a history and do a physical examination. That's what an intern is supposed to do."

"But he doesn't make any sense!" Kenneth whined. "I've been in the room with him for over an hour, and we're still going around in circles. He can't keep the facts straight. I'm frustrated as hell!"

"I'm glad you are honest about it," I said, remembering my own frustrations as a house officer.

Years ago, when I was more committed to the science of medicine than the need to care for frightened humans, I had fought to suppress my anger with people whose anxious confusion frustrated my need to acquire information. I was afraid I might make some dreadful mistake because these terrified people would die without a medication they took at home or, worse, would suffer from an interaction between a new drug and one of their old ones. I found it difficult to avoid being vexed when they described their medications as little white tablets instead of giving them names, because there were about a hundred thousand different kinds of little white tablets. Mellower concerns about frazzled emotions took second place to my anger. I probably made their anxiety worse as I sought to "help" them. They were no less alarmed than I about my potential for making errors if I did not get the facts straight. I learned the hard way that anxiety and the confusion that accompanies it are involuntary.

"Kenneth," I said, "it's not the patients but their anxiety that upsets you. Your patients can't help feeling threatened. We're expected to help them conquer their fears."

"But I don't panic over little things," he said.

"Little things like being helpless in a hospital, being a victim of accidental oversight, or being diagnosed with a bad disease don't look so little when you're the patient. Little moles can look like cancer. Little cancers can look like harbingers of weakness, disability, and death."

"But I've got a job to do," Kenneth said. "I have to take histories and do physical examinations on four patients in the next two hours. I can't spend all my time on one."

I shook my head. I knew how big his task was.

"We must do more than poison cancer cells, Kenneth. Our job is to relieve anxiety as well."

Kenneth is young and strong. He grew up on a farm in western Nebraska. Except for the day he ran his father's combine into a ditch in the middle of the harvest season, I don't think he ever suffered from anxiety. He told me he thought "overly" anxious people were "mental cases."

"I tell them to get a grip on themselves," he said, as if people who *could* get a grip on themselves would spend a single millisecond suffering from this troubling emotion.

Kenneth didn't seem to understand that only a diaphanous curtain of confidence protects each of us from panic. Past experience may raise or lower our threshold or change the nature of the beast that makes us cry for help, but no degree of brute strength can protect us from panic when the appropriate conditions arise.

Some of us panic at the sight of blood, some only when their own blood is spilled. Some cringe in darkened movie houses while watching horror films, while others do not panic unless threatened by live villains.

Given sufficient threats, our minds blow. An elderly widow who screams for the police because she hears an unexplained sound may be no more lacking in courage than the hulking halfback who fears a confrontation with a band of armed thugs. Indeed, it may take considerably more courage for an elderly woman, frail and defenseless, to face the risks of living alone than it does for a two-hundred-pound man to take a stroll at night. A young woman whose serenity is destroyed by a tiny breast cancer is not less courageous than a woman twice her age who smiles confidently when her cancer is "cured" but trembles at the prospect of memory loss. Anxiety afflicts most of us when we are confronted with the prospect of disfigurement, disability, and mortality, our own or that of those we love, no matter how clearly we understand that all humans face similar risks and that death will come to each of us in its own way.

I told Kenneth about Stuart, a physician whom I was asked to see in the hospital on Christmas Day a decade ago. Stuart was frantic when I reached his bedside. With difficulty I helped him piece his history together.

He was forty-two years old and had never previously been ill. Indeed, except for a nagging cough, he had felt completely well until the day he entered the hospital. Two days before Christmas, on a slow day in the office, he decided to have a chest X ray taken. Although he had not had a chest X ray taken for many years, he expected it to be normal because he felt quite well. To his astonishment, the film showed a huge mass in the middle of his chest. Only one explanation seemed to fit the picture: cancer. By his own action the physician had abruptly given himself a fatal diagnosis. Within hours he became irrational. He could not talk in sentences. He could not ask clear questions or pay attention to instructions. He waved away his last patients and retreated into his inner office.

With difficulty, he was able to dial his home telephone number. In a broken voice he explained the problem to his wife. She asked a sitter to care for their children and hurried to the office.

Stuart had not had a physical examination for many years. He had no personal physician. In haste he found a colleague who was willing to admit him to the hospital. Both of them were ill at ease. Both were afraid that Stuart was going to die rather quickly.

I knew Stuart from our work in the hospital. I respected him for his good judgment. Many times we had worked through the night in the intensive care unit, battling to save our patients' lives. We were deliberate in our behavior, relying on the rules of good medicine to carry out our activities. We always maintained our composure as a matter of professional discipline.

When I arrived, I found his wife perched on his bed, stroking his arm while he wept. She struggled to find consoling phrases. He seemed to take no comfort from her presence, almost to reject her soft attentions as an additional irritation.

"I can't understand it," she said. "I've never seen him like this. We've been married for twenty years. What's happening?"

I stayed for hours. Christmas Day was not a holy day for me but a chance to do a good deed by substituting for my colleagues who wished to be with their families. For Stuart, however, the family gathering on Christmas had always been an occasion for joyful anticipation because it was the only day the family spent together, free from other obligations. It was the first Christmas he had ever missed.

I tried to talk with Stuart. But the more I talked, the more restless he became. I felt as if the conversation itself frightened me. He could not understand any medical terms. He could not comprehend ordinary English. Repeatedly, he asked for definitions, then forgot them before I had finished my explanations. He could not fathom the meaning of tests or remember the names of the treatments I told him we might use. One thought alone gripped his attention, the possibility of death.

As much for my own comfort as for his, I held the hope of cure aloft like a golden apple. I felt foolish departing from my consultant's role, seeking to find some means of comforting my patient rather than performing my assigned task. Because of his severe anxiety, we minimized discussion of the issues pertinent to his cancer.

I was able to maintain my professional coolness, even though I could feel my stomach churning. When I looked at Stuart, I saw more than his anxiety. I saw a reflection of myself.

Stuart's anxiety seemed to enlarge as he talked about the crushing effect of his cancer upon his family. Like me, he was proud of his children, the oldest of whom was thirteen. He spoke lovingly about his role in their lives, but his love was overcast with grief.

"That's all over, now," he said, despite my assurances that he had time, real hope, and a good possibility of cure.

As the days passed, Stuart's anxiety dissipated enough to discuss his treatment. I advised aggressive chemotherapy, which had a good chance of cure. He quickly made a decision to take it, becoming almost euphoric in the process.

Stuart was lucky. The treatment cured his cancer. By the following September, he had returned to practice as if he had never been ill. When we pass each other in the halls of the hospital these days, we speak as if the anxiety attack had never occurred. But our relationship has changed. A distance has grown between us. We both survived an awful crisis but from vastly different vantage points. We had both seen the same war, but we had not seen it in the same way.

He never talks about my efforts on that Christmas Day, and about what it meant to him. I doubt he remembers much of it, except that it was horrible to contemplate. I suspect his mental images of the day were dulled by the myriad events that followed in its path, the hellish ordeal of chemotherapy, the uncertainty of survival, and the disruption of his professional life. The memory of the months of testing his mettle as he endured the "treatment" may have provided a powerful antidote to the anxious memories of the day of diagnosis.

I carry an indelible impression of the seemingly endless time I sat at Stuart's bedside, and I remember my helplessness whenever we meet. I never told him about my feelings, my heightened sense of fragility, my awareness that, but for good fortune, I might have been in that hospital bed, fearing for my own life.

My experience with Stuart gave me a frightening glimpse of the thinness of the protective shielding that contains the flames of my emotions.

Just as I cannot always cure anxiety, I cannot always recognize it. I want to hear, but I forget to take the time. I make assumptions when I should ask questions. I trust my own superficial observations when I should probe deeper by listening to my patients' concerns about themselves. I tell people what *I* think instead of asking them what *they* think. And even when they tell me, I don't always listen to their answers. Only later do my errors come home to me. People like Helen reveal my fallibility.

Helen had been my patient for ten years when she came to me with a blister on her foot. I thought I knew Helen quite well by then. She had a thick chart that chronicled decades of disease. She had weathered metastatic breast cancer for eighteen years. She had survived major heart disease. She had undergone repeated back surgery, despite which she walked with difficulty. She had two artificial hips. She had developed brittle, insulin-dependent diabetes at the age of eighty. Yet despite her many ailments, Helen never complained when I asked her how she was.

"As good as can be expected," she would say with a wry grimace.

She faced each new problem with the same tough-minded attitude.

In her younger days Helen had worked in a hospital. She had learned the healing art with its limitations. I felt honored to be her physician. I knew she had fired several others.

For her part, Helen had relished our relationship. She confided in me. Although she was a devout Catholic, I never felt the presence of a religious barrier. Indeed, our shared values helped us bridge such gaps. She sent me cards for every Jewish holy day. In each was a brief message conveying her approval.

As rich as our past relationship had been, it seemed to have little to do with the current problem. Helen's attention was focused on her foot. When I looked at the blister, I did not think much of it. It was almost inconsequential, caused by an ill-fitting shoe.

"My sister died of a heart attack last week," she told me. "I wore the shoe to her funeral." As she told me about the sadness of the day, Helen's voice trembled with an unusual degree of emotion. "Her death was so sudden. She wasn't sick." I knew Helen was aware that death from a heart attack can be sudden.

"I'm glad you came in to let me look at your foot," I said. "We both know foot sores can create serious problems for people who have diabetes. Fortunately, you have nothing to worry about because your blister is quite superficial. Without any treatment it will heal in a few days."

I am embarrassed to admit I said "you have nothing to worry about" to Helen. I suppose it seemed appropriate to me at the time. I reasoned that, if she wasn't anxious about metastatic cancer, severe heart disease, painful arthritis, and brittle diabetes, if she wasn't worried about age itself, the infirmity that accompanied all of her diseases, or the tragedy of watching her siblings pass into the great beyond, the blister should surely be trivial enough to justify indifference to it. I totally forgot that, by its nature, anxiety is irrational and capricious. In fact, our anxiety can easily focus on trivial issues because larger problems are beyond our comprehension. It is easier for me to worry about my serum cholesterol than it is for me to imagine that I might die in a collision.

I am not alone. Isn't our whole population more terrified of Lyme disease than tuberculosis? Don't a few drive-by shootings frighten us more than the thousands of accidental deaths of people shot at home? Doesn't a bomb threat in an elementary school hold our attention more than the threat of destruction of entire cities by urban blight?

Why should Helen's concern about the tiny blister on her foot be proportionate to the threat it created to her life? In fact, she may have found it easier to concentrate her anxiety on the blister precisely because it was *not* a severe threat to her but a curable problem. Her emotional stability may have been rocked by her sister's death. She may have been troubled by the ironic possibility that the blister that she had acquired at her sister's funeral might lead to an amputation of her leg or even her demise. These speculations do little more than titillate the imagination. As her doctor, I had no way of knowing how or why her anxiety level was "disproportionately" raised. In fact, when she left my office, I was so ignorant about Helen that I was unaware that she was still anxious.

Two days later, she consulted another physician without telling me about it. The blister was no worse. The remedy prescribed by the other doctor was the same. But the other doctor did not say, "You have nothing to worry about." The blister healed in a week.

It takes constant vigilance to improve my sensitivity to the concerns of other people about problems that scarcely trouble me at all.

At the opposite extreme from Helen, perhaps, Jean-Louise was plagued with anxiety. Indeed, this fifty-five-year-old woman told me that she had always been a hypochondriac before she developed breast cancer. Her job teaching high school French had been threatened because of her frequent health-related absences. In fact, a month before her mammogram was done, the school superintendent had put her on probation.

When she first came to my office accompanied by her brother, Jean-Louise did not impress me as being overly anxious. Compared to other women who come for their first visit after a breast biopsy, she exhibited the usual degree of concern. She asked many questions. She asked for explanations when she did not understand. I had no reason to expect that anxiety would become her major problem.

Perhaps Jean-Louise took comfort from her brother's presence. Her brother was a forensic pathologist, a physician who did autopsies for the police. He had brought a small notebook in which he jotted down my responses. He rarely spoke.

"We need more studies," I told them.

Within weeks of the abnormal mammogram, we discovered the breast cancer had already spread beyond the lymph nodes in her armpit. A CAT scan of her abdomen revealed two metastases in her liver. We did biopsies to prove they had come from her breast. The biopsies confirmed our suspicion.

I asked her to come back to the office after I obtained the results.

"I didn't know it could spread so quickly," she said.

"It's rare," I said. It would not be the last time rare things happened to Jean-Louise.

"What are you going to do about it?" she asked.

I told her I planned to use chemotherapy.

"Does it ever cure anyone?"

"It produces the appearance of cure. We call it complete remission. If it lasts for several years, complete remission is equivalent to cure in some cancers, like Hodgkin's disease. Unfortunately, complete remissions don't usually last more than a year or two in patients with metastatic breast cancer. I don't believe anyone has ever been cured with chemotherapy."

"No one at all?"

"Well, very few. I don't believe I should promise a cure."

Because there seemed to be no other choice, she started to take chemotherapy the next month. Cautiously, we performed frequent blood tests for signs of liver damage. They were all normal. After a year of treatment, we repeated the CAT scan. The metastases had disappeared.

"The CAT scan isn't perfect, you understand," I told her. "Not all metastases show. I think we should give you more treatment."

"How much?" she asked.

"I don't know," I told her.

We continued the chemotherapy for another year and a half, spacing the doses more widely apart. We could find no evidence of cancer in her liver or anywhere else in her body. Although she looked and felt well, she was filled with doubt.

She came to the office every four weeks, each time complaining of a new lump, most of which were the size of a pinhead or smaller. They were difficult to feel. Each new lump proved to be a tiny thickening of the skin and not a cancerous growth. She would not accept anyone's word but mine on the subject.

Other aspects of her behavior began to disturb me. When I had told her she would probably die from breast cancer in a few years, she seemed to accept my prediction with grim resignation. If the prognosis disturbed her, she never told me about it.

In retrospect, her resignation was possibly related to the facts she repeated many times: her cancer had forced her to lose her job and move from a distant city in order to be nearer to her brother. She had little money, no husband or children, no friends, no hobby, and no diversion. While she taught school, she had befriended many of the students. But she had been unable to maintain any connections with them.

Four years after the breast cancer had disappeared, she noticed a pain in her upper abdomen. The pain varied from mild to intense, especially after dinner. She thought the cancer had returned, but the CAT scan showed no sign of metastases. I examined her often, but could detect no abnormality. Indeed, all her liver tests were normal. I told her I thought we had done enough. Then I went on vacation.

While I was away the pain became much more intense. In agony, she went to an emergency room where doctors quickly detected an acute inflammation of her gall bladder. In fact, it was nearly gangrenous when her surgeon removed it. He took time to examine her liver with his hands while her abdomen was open. There was no sign of cancer.

"You're cured," I said.

"You said it was impossible," she replied.

"I said it was highly unlikely, but I think it happened."

"I find that difficult to believe."

Doubts pestered Jean-Louise like mosquitos humming in a darkened tent. She spent long hours fantasizing about the cancer growing, unseen, in her body.

"That's what it did before we found it the first time," she told me.

She had broken her connections with her home town. Anxiety about her illness prevented her from committing herself to the task of finding a new job. She did not have the emotional strength to work as a tutor or even to volunteer in the schools. I sent her to a psychiatrist.

Together, the psychiatrist and I looked for ways to rehabilitate our patient. It seemed painfully ironic to us both that Jean-Louise, having been cured of cancer, was crippled by the knowledge that she had once had it and the unshakable certainty that it could not be cured. For two years we struggled to rid her of her anxiety. We tried counseling, a support group, activities, and a variety of medications. She made a modest improvement to the point where she would laugh about her troubles with me and deny that she needed further help, but she never became employed or found a strong interest. She spent her days alone in her room, reading or watching television. She was bored with life and waited, impatiently, for it to end.

One Monday morning, about seven years after the diagnosis of metastatic cancer, Jean-Louise appeared in the emergency room. Four days earlier, her brother explained, she had complained of pain on the right side of her chest, a cough, and fever. He believed she had a viral infection and suggested she take cough medicine and aspirin. Although Jean-Louise suspected her problem was much more severe than a viral illness, she did not disclose her suspicions to her brother. Instead, she prepared to die. On Monday morning, when her brother found her languishing in bed, he called the rescue squad.

She was lying on a gurney in the emergency room when I arrived. In hushed tones, the emergency room physician imparted the details of her illness to me. She had a rapid pulse, a low blood pressure, a fever of 103°, and absent breath sounds on the right side of her chest.

"She looks bad," he said.

"Nothing will help me now," Jean-Louise told me in a shaky voice. "The cancer is back. Thank you for everything."

But Jean-Louise's cancer had not come back. A chest X ray soon made it clear that she had pneumonia. Unfortunately, the pneumonia was far advanced. She was in shock. Bacteria grew from her blood. Her kidneys ceased to function. Her extremities turned cool and blue. Despite vigorous efforts to save her, she died.

An autopsy showed no signs of cancer anywhere in her body.

When I first met Jean-Louise, I was not surprised at her severe anxiety. She had a life-threatening cancer, surely a sufficient cause. In the early months of our acquaintance, we busied ourselves with "curing her anxiety by treating her cancer."

Although she had been a chronic hypochondriac before she developed cancer, she had held a job. True, marked absenteeism had created problems with the school system, but it had resulted in a probationary action, not dismissal. From my point of view, anxiety about her health had created a handicap for her rather than a total disability. As she described it, although she visited doctors frequently, she had usually been satisfied with their explanations and returned to work.

When she developed breast cancer, however, her personality seemed to change. She remained edgy, challenging every explanation I gave her, demanding repeated confirmation of earlier reports. It was not unusual for Jean-Louise to call the office several times a day. Although she knew all of the personnel, she would never trust even simple answers unless they came directly from me. She was not quite satisfied to have another physician perform the simplest examination. Only my fingers gave her the assurance she needed to sustain her during her nights of torment while she wondered when and where the dreaded cancer cells would re-emerge in her body.

Most oncologists have had a minimum of psychiatric training. Yet despite our lack of strength in this discipline, we confront powerful emotional disturbances. Experience and sensitivity help oncologists judge which patients should be advised to see psychiatrists. In making such decisions, we can only guess at the severity of our patients' emotional problems and only speculate about the amount of stress that the challenge of psychotherapy may add to their burdens.

Jean-Louise welcomed a referral to a psychotherapist. Yet even with the help of a psychiatrist, she was unable to restore her sense of equilibrium. Her emotional imbalance stemmed from her unhappy childhood.

Jean-Louise was the middle child in a rigid, authoritarian household. Her older brother was brilliant, excelled in school, and later received a full-tuition scholarship to Harvard, graduating with honors. Her younger sister, who was the darling of the family, became the homecoming queen of her high school class. She married a financially successful man and joined a group of women whose lives centered around civic activities, charities, and the local country club. But Jean-Louise was different. She was neither brilliant nor beautiful, studious nor popular, loving, nor beloved. Instead, she was the target of her father's angry disapproval.

Her father, the chief librarian in a small town, had been dismayed by the prophecy of a college English professor.

"You have a weak and lazy brain," the professor had said, after he caught her father plagiarizing a term paper. "You'll never amount to anything in this world."

Within ten years of his college graduation, her father had become heavily dependent on alcohol, consuming several bottles a week.

Often enraged at the dinner table, he singled out Jean-Louise as his target. After one particularly angry attack, Jean-Louise refused to accept any more abuse. At the age of eight, she ceased to speak to her father. Although they lived in the same house for the next fourteen years, she never said a word to him. Even more bizarre than the close-mouthed daughter was the father who failed to notice that he had been excommunicated by his daughter. Yet she maintained her silence until, one night, while he was driving with a bottle of whiskey cradled in his lap, he collided with a lamppost and died. Jean-Louise never wept for him.

A year later, she became engaged to the only boy in her class who had joined the high school Latin club. To avoid the draft, he joined the National Guard and was surprised when he was called to fight in Korea. His body was returned four weeks later. He had been the victim of an accident while training for combat. Jean-Louise never had any romantic interest after that. Although the local high school had given her a secure job teaching French, she had no personal entertainment. She lacked friends, social life, a hobby, or even a pet.

When she was diagnosed with breast cancer, she lost her job. Because her slim savings could not support her, she left the city where she had lived since birth and traveled six hundred miles to live with her brother. Although the move seemed drastic, she depended on his financial support.

Before moving in with him, Jean-Louise had not seen her brother since their mother's funeral, fifteen years earlier. With shock, she realized that her brother looked much more like her father than she remembered. He also appeared to have inherited her father's explosive temper and appetite for alcohol. Like her father, he showed no respect for her. He never asked her opinion or believed her descriptions of her own medical problems. He never found anything nice to say about her.

In short, Jean-Louise suffered from an emotional disorder of long standing. She was as much the victim of a cruel and uncompromising environment as of her inner turmoil. Unfortunately, the emotional disorder was not diagnosed or treated before the cancer was discovered. After the cancer was found, it was too late to help Jean-Louise learn to control her feelings. Instead, she was faced with a series of threatening crises with which she lacked the strength to cope. She had not had an opportunity to develop a means to quench the fires of anxiety. She lacked friends and loved ones who might have served to comfort her. Instead, she faced the terror of cancer and of survival after cancer virtually alone.

Except for her psychiatrist, my office staff, and me, I know of no one who cared for Jean-Louise. Indeed, I think she felt that, except for her fiancé and some of the students she had taught in high school, there never had been.

Friends of anxious people sometimes seize upon the anxiety as if it were a fixable defect. The friends are motivated by an understandable desire to relieve a deep and agonizing pain. Like doctors, they want to *do* something about the symptoms. Like most of us, these friends can recollect an anxious moment of childhood when they were soothed by a caring parent. Soothing can often be accomplished by stroking furry pets or stuffed animals or by feeling a warm human touch. For those of us who have no such memories, who experienced our childhood anxiety in a cold environment, consolation may be much more difficult to obtain.

The anxiety associated with cancer differs from easily soothed childhood fears in a major respect. The source of the fear cannot be easily removed. I suggested psychotherapy to a tremulous, anxious woman, whose anxiety seemed to make her glow like a radiant heater.

"Just cure my cancer, Doctor," she said. "My anxiety will disappear in a second if you do that."

Because I could not cure her cancer, her anxiety remained, destroying any hope she had for comfort in the last years of her life. I sought to relieve what I thought might be a treatable problem, but I never succeeded.

Yet cancer alone does not account for anxiety. Some people never show more than mild levels of it, even when their cancers are life-threatening and return several times. In contrast to people who are terrified of cancer, such individuals rarely dwell on the frightening consequences of malignancy. They take appropriate steps to rid themselves of cancer without appearing to suffer much mental anguish in the process. Such an individual is Jason.

Jason is a retired British diplomat who had spent his younger days traveling in the Caribbean. He had many moles. He was fair-skinned and burned quite easily in the sun, factors that had inconvenienced him during his years in the tropics. Indeed, he had blistered more than once as a result of sun-burn. After moving to Maryland, he had begun to use sunscreen, but it was several decades too late.

He came to me when he discovered a black tumor on his arm. The tumor looked different from the moles. The tumor he showed me measured a little more than half an inch in each direction. It had irregular edges and an uneven coloration. It had a bumpy surface. I knew at once that it was a melanoma, a treacherous skin cancer. Although four out of five people with melanomas are cured by surgery, the rest are plagued by recurrences of the cancer, which may return in the region of the original tumor or spread to distant locations.

"There's only one thing to do," I told Jason. "That is probably a skin cancer and it should be removed."

Jason did not ask many questions. I told him we would know more about the characteristics of the cancer after he had surgery. He smiled as serenely as if he were delivering a suit to the dry cleaner and had been told it would be ready in four days.

"Sounds good to me," he said.

After the surgery, he returned alone for a conference. When I expressed surprise because his wife was not with him, he told me medical information made her nervous.

I told him his melanoma had been moderately deep. Although we could see no sign of spread, there was a distinct possibility that the cancer would come back. If it spread beyond his arm, it would probably be fatal.

"All we can do is hope," he said.

I agreed with him. Although many treatments had been tried, only surgery had been established as a curative treatment for melanoma.

Jason returned every three months for physical examinations. Each time I palpated his arm and axilla with particular care, since this was the area at greatest risk for recurrence. We talked about the possibility that the cancer might return. He never questioned me deeply, never raised a tense eyebrow, never asked me to repeat anything I had said.

I thought perhaps he believed in his own invincibility. Not wishing to dampen his hopes, I did nothing to dissuade him. I could see no harm in letting him ignore the possibility that the melanoma might come back. Yet I bore the knowledge that each trip to my office could mean the end of the comfort of the "complete remission" his surgeon had given him.

After two years of repeated examinations, Jason found a pea-sized lump in his armpit. He made an appointment, more casually than I expected. He appeared in my office, unhurried.

"What do you think it is?" he asked.

"I think it's a lump," I said. "And since it wasn't there before and it is now, it is almost certainly a cancer, probably a melanoma."

"What should we do about it, old chap?"

"Have it removed."

Jason returned a week after the surgeon had removed the lump. As he sat down in my office, I stared at the biopsy report. The pea-sized lump had indeed been a melanoma. I expected him to be despondent when I told him the sad news.

"Well, I'm glad it's gone," he said.

"Yes," I said soberly in my prepared-to-listen voice. I rocked back in my chair and waited.

"I mean it's done with," he said.

"You are aware of the possibility that it could come back again."

"Of course I am, Doctor. You've seen to that. There's nothing else to do now though, is there?"

We returned to our three-month ritual, in the hope that whatever melanoma came back could be removed with curative intent. Because hope was all Jason and I could count upon, we treated it like a mutual friend.

Throughout the next two years, I never saw Jason act nervous or concerned. He asked about my family. I inquired about his. We often chatted about friends in the neighborhood. Occasionally, I made sly references to the regular appearance of the royal family in the *National Enquirer*, and he laughed heartily at my innuendoes. I found it impossible to detect any sign of concern.

"Maybe he's right," I thought, finding it difficult to believe myself. "Maybe he is the lucky one, and the melanoma is never coming back again."

I should have bitten my tongue. On the next visit, there was another pea-sized lump on the top of his right shoulder.

"Do you suppose this is another one?" he asked.

It was as if he had found a pokeweed in his garden. A nuisance, nothing more.

"They don't hurt at all, you know," he said.

"You're right," I said. "They don't hurt when they're under the skin but they are dangerous. Let's have it removed."

When he returned after the third surgery for melanoma, still calm, still cheerful, still inquiring politely after my children, it was hard for me to contain my curiosity. The twinkle in his eye encouraged me to ask him how he managed to remain so calm.

"I am at peace," he said.

"What is your secret?"

"I'm not a worrier," he said. "Never have been. If something can be done about a problem, I do it. If it can't, I accept it. We've done everything we could about the melanoma. Now I've got to attend to my garden and repair my porch. I'm not getting younger, you know."

"I understand you, Jason. Yet I am still confused. How do you manage to avoid feeling worried?"

"There's one very good reason why I never worry. It never helps me feel better or get the job done."

"Perhaps you had an experience long ago that made your current challenges seem less important?"

"None of that."

I am unable to explain Jason's lack of anxiety, his acceptance of his cancer. He said he had always lived in the present, never been inclined to elaborate, exaggerate, or speculate. He never missed an appointment, never failed to inquire about the laboratory tests, never ignored the consequences of his malignancy. Yet his level of tension never seemed to rise, and I doubt his friends knew he had cancer three times.

Worry does not help us conquer insuperable difficulties. In fact, I suspect that excessive worry prevents us from taking effective action when we should. When our worry grows to massive anxiety, when it shifts to raw, incoherent terror about unseen or imagined threats or monstrous, unacceptable, but inescapable perils, there is no question that we are ineffective. Yet even when we think we are being reasonable, when logical questions flow freely through our mildly troubled brains, we find ourselves much like Hamlet in his reverie, mulling about present and future miseries. Such a state of mind "puzzles the will, and makes us rather bear those ills we have than flee to others that we know not of."

Hamlet did not choose to be a worrier. I can't prove it, but I don't think he liked worrying. I think he could not help it. I, too, am a worrier. Indeed, many of my patients encourage me to worry about them. Often that means that they can worry less about themselves. I believe my worrying fuels my energy as a professional. Indeed, I call my worries "concerns," but I don't fool anyone when I do it. My patients read my emotions in my body language. A tense eyebrow, a hurried cough, an inappropriate joke, even an averted gaze means more than speech to my patients.

On one occasion, a minor problem caused me to worry about my own health. The day had started innocently. I went out to fetch the paper at the end of the front walk as I do every morning. I bent down to grab it, and when I straightened up, I realized that I had double vision. I was certain that the problem had started suddenly. I wondered what had happened and whether it would disappear. I walked into the house and started to make some coffee.

While I ate breakfast, I tried to read the newspaper. The double vision persisted. I had difficulty making out the fine print. I tried covering my eyes, one at a time, and made an even more startling discovery. The left eye was fine. I had double vision in my right eye. I could see two overlapping images.

Far from believing I know everything about medicine, I am keenly aware of the limitations of my knowledge in many areas, especially ophthalmology. Aside from being able to identify my eye problem as monocular diplopia, I was certain of only one thing: double vision in one eye was a sign of hysteria. Yet I had no clear reason to think I was suffering from hysteria. I had not even glanced at the front page of the newspaper with its daily cargo of wanton murder, avaricious fraud, and the lascivious dalliances of prominent politicians.

As a physician accustomed to solving difficult problems, I did the rational thing, of course. I went to work and acted as if nothing were wrong. Was this a lack of worry? I would prefer to call it inertia. After all, I had a full schedule of patients who were expecting me to see them. I knew that I might have canceled my appointments if it were absolutely necessary, but there seemed no point to it. I did not feel sick. I had no pain. I certainly didn't want to humiliate myself by taking time off from work to be told I was hysterical for *claiming* that I had double vision in one eye when intelligent doctors all knew that it was physically impossible. Because of my embarrassment, I told no one about my problem.

By eleven o'clock I began to have second thoughts about my approach to my diplopia. For one thing, I found it difficult to examine people with my right eye, particularly because my right eye is the dominant one. I could manage to peer into the ears with my left eye, but when I looked into my patients' right pupils with my left eye our noses touched.

"Isn't something a little different?" asked a gentleman after briefly sharing his bristly moustache with me.

I decided to call my ophthalmologist. I wanted an immediate explanation and an instant cure.

"We can give you an appointment in six weeks," I was told.

I wondered why my ophthalmologist wanted me to wait six weeks to see him.

"How about yesterday?" I asked. "Can I see him yesterday?" I was mildly disappointed at the coolness of his receptionist's response.

"Well, I could give you an appointment at the end of the day," she said. "I didn't realize it was urgent."

I began to entertain fantasies about my eye. I looked in a few of my medical books. Monocular diplopia was not listed.

"I can't be making this up," I said to myself, but my certainty was on the wane.

I wondered if I were going blind. I read about the symptoms of retinal detachment, concerned that my condition might represent a variant. Nothing remotely like it was mentioned.

"Perhaps it's a rare manifestation," I thought and began to worry about that possibility.

New thoughts occurred to me. Perhaps there was a problem in my central nervous system, a malfunction in the back of my brain. I considered the possibility of a brain tumor. That would be ironic, but it could explain the rarity of my problem and the difficulty I had finding descriptions of it under "Eye Diseases."

"I told you it was all in your head, you idiot," I said to myself, but reading through the chapters on neurology, I found no mention of the symptom. After searching through three textbooks and coming up empty-handed, I felt more humiliated at my ignorance. After what seemed like endless hours, I finished with my last patient and headed to the ophthalmologist's.

I found my attitude changing as I drove into his parking lot. My "white coat" personality disappeared. I wanted to be his patient, not his colleague. I wanted him to explain everything to me in detail. I wanted to be returned to perfect health. I wanted my problem to be both obvious and curable. I desperately did *not* want him to tell me that it was all in my imagination.

In one sense I *was* treated like a patient when I arrived. I was handed a form to fill out and then another and another.

"I'd rather pay cash than apply for a mortgage," I joked.

The receptionist did not even grin.

To busy myself, I picked up a magazine I would never otherwise have read. I flipped through the journal without appreciating its contents. Repetitious thoughts about my eyesight distracted my attention. I felt self-conscious as I covered my right eye to read.

I glanced around the room. The other patients seemed to have difficulty reading, too. Their sad faces and sagging shoulders made me aware of their discomfort. A doctor's waiting room can be depressing.

Soundlessly, the nurse appeared. I heard my name spoken in a whisper. I marched after her down a tiled hallway with many doors. She showed me into a darkened room and asked me to be seated in a mechanical throne. I was surrounded by equipment which looked more suited to a planetarium than a physician's office. I expected Dr. Golden to appear at once, but no one came for several minutes. Then the soundless nurse returned without the doctor. She asked me to read from a card.

"I can't read with my right eye," I said. "That's why I'm here."

"Read it anyway," she said, coldly. "We need it for our records."

I felt a sense of déjà vu. I had often said the same thing to my own patients. Documentation has come to define my medical practice. I am not satisfied when I focus my attention on my patients' complaints. If I haven't recorded information, I cannot prove I have obtained it.

"When did your difficulty begin?" she asked.

I told her about my problem while I wondered if Dr. Golden would ever hear my version of the story in the words I had so carefully chosen. Perhaps some little detail the nurse might omit would clarify the problem for him.

I recalled my own patients saying to me, "It's not a pain, really. It's more like an ache, a deep ache." I always note their exact words, although the distinctions they have made often mean nothing to me.

With the roles reversed, I found myself emphasizing words,

time sequences, and degrees of severity as if the diagnosis depended on them.

"My complaint is simple," I said. "I see double from my right eye. One object is a fraction of an inch above the other."

"I didn't know that was possible," the nurse said. I sensed rejection in her voice.

"Well it is!" I said more hotly than I intended.

"It must be, if you say so, Doctor!" she said, emphasizing my title. She sounded hostile but submissive. Indeed, I could imagine her acquiescing in the same deferential tones if I had insisted that the sun went round the earth. I was relieved when she left.

"What have we here, Daniel?" Dr. Golden asked. His voice sounded strangely different from the one he used when we encountered each other in the halls of the hospital. I felt a distance in it I could not explain. It was as if he, too, were ready for some disaster.

For an instant, anxious thoughts sped through my mind. Perhaps some dire illness, unrecognized by me, was obvious to him. Maybe he was afraid to tell me the awful news that I would die or be disabled. If I had a brain tumor, he would not want to claim the credit for finding it. Instead of telling him my fears, I made a joke about his Porsche and my Vega. He did not laugh.

"Did the nurse tell you my history?" I asked, simultaneously reluctant to waste his time with repetition and fearful lest he miss some vital piece of information. "I'm afraid she thinks I'm nuts."

"Let's have a look," he said, avoiding a direct response to my comment.

While the glowing light from his ophthalmoscope seemed to glare into the recesses of my brain, I wondered if he, too, doubted my sanity. Perhaps my double vision was an early sign of shell shock. Time for a vacation, I thought.

Imposed between me and Dr. Golden was a complex, expensive-looking piece of equipment, an instrument composed of intricate devices suspended on hinged arms with which he attacked my eye. I had never been examined with such intensity. Although he used a topical anesthetic to numb my eyeball, I had to force myself to hold still. I felt nauseated and vaguely alarmed throughout the examination, but I said nothing.

Dr. Golden studied me in silence, pausing occasionally to jot notes on a sheet of paper attached to a clipboard. I could see he was writing in my chart, but I dared not ask what he had found.

When he was finished with the examination, he left the room. As I waited for him to return, thoughts flitted through my brain like moths bouncing around a lone light bulb after dark. I wondered if surgery would be required, or an eye patch. I wondered if I would be disabled for days, weeks, months, or possibly forever.

Dr. Golden returned with his associate. His calm demeanor seemed even more forced than it had been before.

"Take a look at this, Jeff," he said.

I did not want to be a museum object, to have something rare that no one ever sees except in textbooks of strange diseases. Had he found some bizarre anomaly, like a loa loa worm, doing a dance across my conjunctival sac? We giggle when, as medical students, we first learn about weird medical problems. I don't think it's at all funny to have them.

My wife has a strange disease of the eye. Her doctor found it when she was a teenager.

"In twenty years I've never actually seen a case," her doctor had told her at the time, "but it looks like a textbook picture." The rare event meant threatened blindness for my wife. She had spent months in a research hospital before the disease remitted, leaving her with a blind spot. Had I acquired my wife's ailment?

"I see what you are talking about," the associate said. If anything, his voice was flatter than Dr. Golden's. "I think it's benign." They exchanged a few comments I did not understand, and then Dr. Golden thanked him, and the associate left the room. After an annoying silence, during which my fantasies reached their zenith, he spoke directly to me.

"You have two findings in that eye, Daniel," Dr. Golden said at last. "The problem which brought you here is trivial. It's called central retinal edema. It will disappear in a few days whether we treat it or not. Prednisone will make it go away a little faster, and

I'll be happy to prescribe it. The other problem is either a benign variant or a malignant growth on the iris. I don't have to tell you that cancers of the iris are quite rare. Since I've never seen your eye before, I have no basis for comparison. I'd like you to come back in six weeks so that I can check it again."

"But is my double vision going to improve?"

"In a day or two, I think."

I felt a deep sense of appreciation, as if I had been given an answer to an unspoken prayer. I wanted to pay Dr. Golden in order to show my appreciation. Clutching my prednisone prescription, I stopped at his front desk where the soundless nurse sat, sorting through insurance forms.

"How much will it be?" I asked.

"You're a doctor," she said.

"And therefore, I can afford to pay. How much will it be?"

"Dr. Golden doesn't charge doctors," she said.

I felt deeply disappointed at my inability to show my gratitude. I felt as if he had returned my precious sight to me and I owed him something in return. His courteous behavior did not relieve my sense of indebtedness.

A glow suffused my face as I drove back to my office to finish the day's work. The staff was gone, but my partners were still at their desks. None of them knew about my symptom or my concern. Confident that I would be cured, I told them the story, hesitating as I neared the end.

"What was it?" one of them asked. "What was the diagnosis?"

I looked at them strangely, then started laughing.

"You're not going to believe this," I said.

"Try us."

"Well, I can't remember what he said. All I know is that it was a big, long word and it wasn't serious."

I never told anyone about the growth on my iris. When I went back for the follow-up visit, Dr. Golden decided it was indeed benign, and I ceased to think about it.

6
ANGER

There are no "good" or "bad" people.
Some are a little better or a little worse but all are
activated more by misunderstanding than malice.
A blindness to what is going on in each other's hearts.
—Tennessee Williams, quoted by
Elia Kazan in *A Life* (1988)

ANGER is a devilish emotion. It distorts our personalities, turns us into monsters. When we are overcome with anger, even our sweet smiles cannot conceal our degradation. We feign a dignified bearing, but anger controls our thoughts. We seek sympathy from others; often they give it to us. Meanwhile, we are obsessed with a desire to hurt, harm, or destroy.

Anger changes our internal environment. It makes our faces flush, our pupils dilate, our hearts race, and our breathing accelerate. It also causes sweating, increases stomach acid, and makes muscles tense. Angry people grind down their teeth, develop heart disease and ulcers, hypertension and hemorrhoids. Angry nations wage war. As an emotion of the primitive, anger helps to insure survival. In the context of civilization, we must ask ourselves how best to handle our anger.

Cancer readily provokes anger. Most of us, patients and families, doctors and medical staffs, work hard to control our anger. But despite our efforts, we often lose the battle. When cancer attacks us or those we care about, it will kindle our rage. Sometimes cancer will make us disproportionately angry about a clogged drain or a flat tire. At other times we will scream at a physician or a nurse or someone we love dearly. Our rage at cancer can make us furious with people on the sidelines, like clerks, housekeepers, dieticians, billing agents, and answering services. The admonition to calm down is usually no more effective than the advice to stop worrying.

People expect oncologists to be "used to it," but I don't believe our anger disappears with practice. After a day of tending my many patients with cancer, their families, and my staff, a day in which I have responded to massive pain, enormous grief, and insurmountable frustration, I've often caught myself raging at a busy signal on the telephone.

I have made the mistake of assuming that my anger about cancer can be eliminated by self-control. With great effort I have concealed my rage behind a mask of pleasantness and even joviality. But like a caged panther, my anger has paced back and forth, growling, waiting for an opportunity to escape and find a victim. I'm fortunate when the victims are tennis balls.

"Anyone but Dr. Starch!" Toby said.

"I beg your pardon?" I asked.

"You said you wanted a lung specialist to look at me. I don't want Dr. Starch."

I was surprised at Toby's statement. In the two months since I had begun to care for him, I had never seen him angry, never heard him say a cross word. But his fury at Dr. Starch was unmistakable.

Toby had pneumonia. I expected it to clear rapidly with antibiotics, but I wanted reassurance from a lung specialist. Dr. Starch was the logical choice. He knew Toby. He had studied his lungs and diagnosed his cancer. If any problems developed, Dr. Starch would be prepared to respond because of his familiarity with Toby's history. Although I knew that other pulmonary doctors could care for him, they would feel less comfortable than Dr. Starch.

"I don't mind," I said. "But why do you want another specialist? Dr. Starch is excellent."

Toby's face turned bright red.

"I like you, Doctor. I don't want to make trouble for you. But our family is furious at Dr. Starch. He missed the diagnosis in July. His partner scared us to death in January. Why shouldn't I be angry at him?"

Toby's anger decided the issue.

People often ask why they shouldn't be angry, as if an angry response was most appropriate when someone else makes an "error." The question sounds logical. Many accept without question the premise that "people should be more careful, especially doctors."

How could I persuade Toby that Dr. Starch had not made an "error"? Although he "missed" the diagnosis, Dr. Starch had followed all the appropriate steps for evaluating a suspicious cough. It was not his "fault" that the tumor was beyond the reach of his instruments.

Toby's question dogs my profession: "Why shouldn't I be angry? My doctor didn't. . . . " or "My doctor did . . . " Yet the constant opportunities for people to be angry with us as we practice medicine staggers the imagination. We cannot work without making "errors" like the one Dr. Starch made or worse. Occasionally our fingers slip, our eyes miss details, our ears hear incorrectly, our equipment malfunctions, our tests don't work; our judgments, which are the product of our use of all these things, cannot meet the expectations of a public mesmerized by the wonders of technology, hopeful that we doctors will be perfect.

Why shouldn't our patients be angry? Because their anger fuels their desire to attack other people. Because their anger distracts them from fighting to survive. Because their anger does not correct the problem.

Although I believed Toby's anger was harmful to him, I could not help him quell it. I was afraid to comment about his anger lest I feed it and make a bad situation worse. Toby appeared too fragile. Dr. Starch could survive being fired.

Dr. Starch and I had worked together for many years. He was careful, conscientious, self-confident, and self-effacing. As a physician, he was an ideal role model. He showed concern for people. He spoke in soft but measured tones. He loved his work. Patients and other doctors thought highly of him.

My knowledge of Dr. Starch made Toby's outburst seem rash. But Toby had not spent years learning to trust Dr. Starch as I had. He had not spent nights with him in the emergency room battling to save lives. He had not pored over charts and X-rays with him, looking for clues to help unravel complex problems. Without hesitancy I would have trusted Dr. Starch with my life, not because I was certain he could succeed, but because I don't think anyone else could have done better.

Ironically, although they could not share their feelings with each other, both Dr. Starch and Toby had been hurt by the "missed" diagnosis. Toby told his friends about it. They shared his disappointment and his anger.

No one listened to Dr. Starch. He tried to tell his wife, but she said, "What did you expect? You're a doctor. Things like that happen." Then she changed the subject.

Gradually, as Toby repeated his story, his anger began to build. Anxious friends asked Toby if his cancer might not have been cured if it had been diagnosed earlier. He fended off their insinuations; he knew Dr. Starch had done his best. But as time went on, he felt more hostile towards him.

I felt torn. Loyal to both, I wanted to find some way to reunite them. Unresolved anger hurt them both. But the hour was late, the issue elusive, the chance of reconciliation remote. Reluctantly, I agreed to find another pulmonary specialist.

Within days the pneumonia cleared. To our mutual relief, Toby was well enough to go home.

Anger adds to cancer's burden. Indeed, for Sadie, a seventy-two-year-old woman with cancer, anger caused more suffering than her malignancy.

Sadie had one cancer in her pelvis, a second in her lung. Her oncologist was fascinated with the accidental event of two different malignancies occurring simultaneously in the same patient. He was at pains to develop a chemotherapeutic regimen for her. Sadie wasn't interested. She wanted relief from pain. She complained incessantly, and when the oncologist ignored her pleas, she fired him. I met him later at the nursing station.

"It's about time someone else took over," he told me. "I can't get her attention. I tried to talk to her about the cancer in her chest, and she only wanted to talk about her back pain. I know her back hurts. I've done everything I could to relieve her back pain. But that's not life-threatening. The cancer in her lung could be fatal. Maybe you can get her to listen to reason."

Sadie's daughter, Bunny, had asked me to supervise her mother's care. She said her mother would be delighted to see me, but Sadie only scowled. Sadie would not discuss her back pain or her cancers. To all specific questions about her physical condition she responded with a string of complaints about doctors, nurses, clerks, and aides, about bills and medications, about humiliations and insults. She was not content with general references to the injuries other people had caused her but flooded me with detailed information. As a result, despite her daughter's encouragement, I found it difficult to acquire any medically useful information about her.

Sadie ignored the efforts I made on her behalf. Because of her impatience with the other oncologist, I made a special trip to visit her. Her long discourse caused me to keep patients waiting in my office. Despite her anger she failed to give me clues as to how I might help her. Rather than learn about problems I could solve, I heard about past injuries I could not relieve. I struggled to maintain my self-control.

Because I wanted to help her, I ignored my restless urge to withdraw from Sadie. Instead, I listened to all of her complaints. I hoped to elicit her cooperation by displaying interest in her one-sided wars.

Jack, her husband, hovered in the corridor, barely out of earshot. He approached me after I left the room. Although my cheeks burned after listening to his wife's rage, I dug deep to find some kind feelings for him.

"It's best not to ask her specific questions," he told me. "She can't take it."

"I got the message," I said. "I'll do everything I can to help her feel better. I'll need all the help you can give me."

As her cancer enlarged and spread, her monologues grew angrier and included everyone. She did not spare me, her husband, or her children. She ignored the sacrifices we made to be with her. Her daughter, Bunny, relinquished her vacation time and asked her children to cook for themselves so she could remain at her mother's side. But Sadie shook an enraged finger in her face.

"Get out of here!" she said. "I never want to see you again."

I happened to be on the scene as Bunny left the room. She choked back her tears. I grasped her hand for a moment, seeking strength besides delivering it. Then I entered Sadie's room.

"I don't know what's wrong with me," Sadie said.

I gave her time to talk. She described her anger with the nurses.

"They don't treat me with respect!" she said. "They don't seem friendly."

When we spoke of the possibility that she might die, however, she smiled blandly as if it did not concern her.

"I've got cancer, don't I?" she said.

Later, at the nursing station, I grappled with the problem of explaining Sadie's behavior to the staff. I tried to find a context in which her anger could be seen as a symptom of disease rather than bad behavior. I wanted them to view Sadie's incessant demands with professional detachment, to monitor her angry outbursts as they would a fever, her nagging criticisms as if they were her pains.

The nurses accepted Sadie's anger better than I did. Whatever its explanation, they had learned to cope with it. Their survival as nurses hinged on their ability to respond to anger with gentle reassurance.

I tried to understand her casual attitude toward death and disability, her intense anger about the hospital food and the regulation of the air conditioner. Just as I could more easily scream at a busy signal than I could at cancer, Sadie asked God to punish the people who cared for her but gracefully accepted her impending death.

Because Sadie could not come to me, I went to her. Her medical problems were beyond cure. Because her cancer did not respond to chemotherapy, I discontinued it. I had little to offer besides nourishment, physical therapy, pain control, and my time. So I listened to her complaints each time I visited, in the belief that my listening might ease her misery.

When she died, I received a lovely thank-you note from Bunny.

Although Sadie was a challenge to us, we could cope because she was confined to bed. In addition, her family understood the inappropriate nature of her rage. We do not cope as well with angry patients who are more active and whose families share their fury. Then all involved are at risk of becoming sensitive, distant, even hostile. It is easier for me to comfort a raging patient than it is to provide solace to an angry friend or relative. The basis of my difficulty, I suppose, is the relationship itself. The patient has engaged my services. Moreover, I have access to information, sometimes closely guarded secrets, to help me understand the roots of my patient's anger. The friends and relatives are not my patients. I see only open mouths hurling epithets, commanding fingers held on high. I cannot see the pain deep inside where the fury burns furnace-hot.

Raging relatives do not become angry with the world simply because someone they love has cancer. People who rage about cancer usually have many other unresolved issues that anger them.

But in a doctor's office, where time is precious, we often miss the larger picture.

Jeb and his wife, Tina, looked angry when I first met them. Jeb stared at me from beneath ridged eyebrows. He growled when he talked about his medical history. Tina's eyes looked everywhere except at mine. Hatred suffused her face.

Not until later did I learn they both had survived angry divorces. Their brief marriage to each other had been an oasis of pleasure after years of unhappiness. Yet because our main concern was treatment of his lung cancer, I knew none of this when they first came to see me.

Jeb had come to me for treatment. I had given him an early appointment and ushered him into my office as soon as they arrived. Tina followed. I could not conceive a reason for their anger. Yet their irritation made me uneasy. I urged them to talk about it.

"I'm not any more upset than I should be," Jeb said. "The doctor told me I am going to die."

"Six weeks to three months was all he gave him," Tina added.

I looked startled.

"We *asked* him how long," she said. "He wasn't going to tell us. We insisted. We *had* to know."

I did not ask them why.

"Did the doctor offend you?"

"No, doctor. Look, we're not angry. Let's just get on with it, shall we?" Tina said. "If we've only got a few months left, we don't want to waste them."

I felt excluded. For me to ignore their anger while talking about Jeb's cancer was impossible. How could I overlook feelings that hovered so near the surface? It was an unreasonable request, but I agreed.

I learned that Jeb, a fifty-one-year-old attorney, had no previous illnesses. In April he decided to give up his two-pack-a-day smoking habit in order to buy a life insurance policy. In May he developed an irritating cough, which antibiotics failed to cure. His doctor treated him by telephone. Unfortunately, Jeb's cough worsened. He became short of breath.

Alarmed about his breathing, Jeb switched doctors. A chest X-ray showed a density in his right lung. The doctor interpreted it as pneumonia. Another course of antibiotics failed to clear the infection. Jeb was sent to Dr. Carver, a lung specialist.

"You have fluid in your chest," Dr. Carver told Jeb, confident that the fluid had been caused by the pneumonia. "It's called a pleural effusion. We'll have to remove it."

The fluid contained cancer cells, as did specimens Dr. Carver obtained from Jeb's right lung. After he made the diagnosis, Dr. Carver had talked about treatment options. He answered detailed questions. He held nothing back. He advised Jeb to consult a radiation therapist and me.

Although they appeared angry, they insisted they were not. In fact, they never quarreled with my staff or me. But their fury gleamed like fire. The contractions of their jaw muscles rippled in the hollows of their cheeks.

The weekend before the chemotherapy was to begin, Jeb developed a painful left calf. I examined it and decided he had phlebitis, inflammation of a vein. His physician ordered tests and treatment for it.

I was surprised when his physician called me shortly before they were due to arrive in my office for a scheduled appointment.

"I was only fifteen minutes late, but they were furious," he said. "I can't believe it. I had an emergency at the hospital. They arrived at my office at 9:00 AM, and I got there at 9:15. They were boiling over. I couldn't understand it. They knew where I had been. Her rage eclipsed his. I suggested psychotherapy. She treated my suggestion as an insult.

"By the way, Jeb's phlebitis is better. You can go ahead with the chemotherapy."

Amongst our colleagues we physicians consider ourselves each other's equals. An unwritten law bars us from criticizing each other because we dare not intimate that we possess a talent, skill, or special gift that sets us over other physicians. Yet even so, I wondered at the casual way in which the doctor had suggested psychotherapy to an enraged woman. Did he believe his suggestion would be followed? Or was it likely to further aggravate her?

If brief delays enraged the couple, I doubted they would be happy in my waiting room. A fifteen-minute wait is not unusual. In fact, a longer delay is common, as my patients are allowed to extend their time with me until they feel finished. Most of my patients have encouraged me in this practice even if it keeps me from conforming to a rigid schedule. I suspected Jeb and Tina would not be pleased with this arrangement. Fortunately, I was able to bring them into my office exactly at the time of his appointment. When they were seated, I told them I had heard from Jeb's physician.

"The nerve of him!" Tina erupted. "I told him to apologize for keeping us waiting. I wanted him to say he was sorry. But instead he told me I needed therapy. I don't like being told I need therapy by someone who is rude and keeps me waiting. Time is precious to us. Jeb had to miss a half day of work to make that appointment. I don't know why we had to see two doctors in one day."

"You sound angry," I said.

"Well, I *am* angry," she shouted, looking directly at me for the first time. "The man is a jackass. I happen to be in therapy. What difference does that make? I handle my problems with my therapist. I still don't see why I should be kept waiting. It happens that my therapist is out of town this week. That doesn't give him the right to be rude to me."

The needs of angry people with cancer sometimes becloud their awareness of the needs of others. The urgency associated with fatal illness distorts their vision, making them lose sight of the conflicting responsibilities of their physicians. Even so, it is remarkable how gracious many people with cancer can be in allowing the needs of others to take precedence over their own.

"It wasn't deliberate," I said carefully, mindful that an upsurge of anger might be in the offing.

"You don't understand," Tina said. "Jeb works constantly. Fifteen minutes is important to him."

"Work is my life," Jeb said. He then proceeded to elaborate.

Although I perceived him as a moderately sick man, who breathed heavily when at rest, he told me he was working six days a week on a report due in a few months. He gave the date. Somewhere in my mental microprocessor a circuit closed. The report was due the week of his anticipated demise.

"No time for Tina?" I asked, raising an eyebrow. With time running out, I found his obsession with work somewhat puzzling.

"They made me acting chief of the department," Jeb told me with a gleam in his eye. "If I work another three years, I'll get double the pension. My retirement fund will be more than ample for Tina's needs."

Three years! I wondered if I should disabuse him. How many times did he need to be reminded? My guess: none.

"You know how Congress is," she said. "They want the report before the end of the session. The White House is in on it, too."

They explained that Jeb had become acting chief the week before the cancer had been diagnosed. No one else could furnish the report before the deadline. Jeb liked to work, took his responsibilities seriously. Languishing at home seemed worse than death to him.

Confident I understood the source of their anger, I called his physician to describe my findings.

"Time is precious to them both. She wants more time with him, and he feels he has to work. I think that was what made the fifteen minutes seem so important," I said.

Jeb's cancer responded to chemotherapy. His chest X-ray looked much improved. Two months later, he was back in my office, however. He looked pale and short of breath. He could barely walk upstairs.

"There is fluid in your right chest cavity," I told him. "It should be tapped again. I'll send you back to Dr. Carver."

I called the specialist, arranged for a tap the same afternoon, and sent Jeb and Tina to his office.

Later that evening, Dr. Carver called me.

"You didn't tell me about their anger," he said.

I braced myself for the next line.

"After I did the tap, I asked Jeb to have another chest X-ray. I wanted to exclude an air leak. They were asked to wait for fifteen minutes while the technician finished with another patient. They left my office. The technician called their house. They were at home, watching television.

"I wasn't hurt by their anger, of course. It's like water off a duck's back. But I don't understand it. Why would he rather sit in his house than in my waiting room?"

The next day, Jeb returned to my office for another round of chemotherapy. After examining Jeb, I broached the subject of their angry departure from Dr. Carver's office.

"First of all," Jeb said, "Their charges are outrageous. Their billing procedures are ridiculous, their business office is an obscenity. We were pushed around from one part of their office to another. When they told us to wait until they were ready for us, I figured it was time to go. My life is too short to waste time in their office. Besides, I had already had one chest X-ray. I didn't need to have two in one day."

"He had a reason for ordering the second chest X-ray," I said. "He wanted to exclude an air leak. I don't know about his charges, but perhaps you could ask him. I've had bills from my plumber that were higher than Dr. Carver's."

"This isn't a joking matter, Doctor."

I was sorry to hear him say that. I am always more hopeful if people can laugh about their troubles.

"But isn't there some way we can learn to deal with these situations without having an outburst?" I asked. "I want to help you in any way I can, but when you express your anger in their offices, the doctors and their staffs are offended. If you continue to make your feelings known, it will be difficult for us to arrange needed treatments."

"So it's our problem, is it!" Tina said. "They run a lousy office, push us around, make us wait, and it's our problem because we tell them we don't like it. Who is all this service supposed to be for?"

"I'm sorry," I said. "I didn't mean to offend you. Of course, the service is for you and your husband. I find doctors' offices uncomfortable, unpleasant places myself. I suspect it's even harder when you have an unpleasant reason for being there. You would rather not see an oncologist or have a tube put into your chest or be told you're getting worse. Yet there you are, not only with an appointed time to do it but the additional burden of waiting past that time because the doctor is late. And it doesn't make you feel any better to be told that the doctor is with other patients who have similar needs.

"The situation is enough to aggravate anyone. But I still believe it is better to control your anger. Angry outbursts make bad situations worse. When people feel your anger, they react to it."

"Don't patronize me," Tina said, her eyes blazing.

"I didn't mean to," I said. "I thought I was being sympathetic."

"I don't need your sympathy."

"Fair enough," I said. "But I wanted to let you know that I hear your reasons for being angry with Dr. Carver's office. I just don't think another office could do any better."

"As long as he's competent, we'll use him," Jeb said. "We'll do whatever it takes to get the job done. But we don't have to like it."

Two weeks later, after his second course of chemotherapy, Jeb had another chest X-ray taken. The cancer had shrunk to less than half its original size. Jeb's appetite had improved. He had not missed a day of work. The report he had been writing would be finished no more than five days beyond the deadline. His work had received high praise from his department chief. I had hoped Jeb would be jubilant, but he looked depressed.

"What's wrong?" I asked.

"Nothing," he replied. "I just don't feel good."

Tumor shrinkage, the hallmark by which chemotherapeutic "success" is usually measured, had not improved his quality of life. His appetite had improved, his face looked pinker, and his breath sounded less strained. But the chemotherapy had made his muscles weak. He had no energy.

After four courses of chemotherapy, I arranged to do a CAT

scan. If the cancer had shrunk, we planned to continue therapy; if the cancer had enlarged, we planned to stop it. I asked Jeb and Tina to come to my office with his films.

"It's exactly the same size," I said when we examined them together. "I don't think the cancer has grown, but it certainly isn't going away."

We talked about the various options, including radiation therapy and chemotherapy. When we were finished, I noticed the look of weariness on their faces.

"It's been a long day," I said.

"You don't know the half of it," Tina told me.

"What do you mean?"

"Jeb's mother died this morning."

They had not told me she was ill.

"She's been unable to eat for eight months. When she was in the hospital, the doctor decided she had cancer. He told us that it was too far gone to pursue, that the stress of surgery would kill her. We took her home. Until Jeb discovered he had cancer, we took care of her. Afterwards, Jeb's fifteen-year-old niece took over. We've been worried ever since."

"About your mother?"

"About our niece, Jenny. Suppose her grandmother died while Jenny was alone with her. She's very sensitive. It would have been a miserable experience."

"Was Jenny close to your mother?"

"Extremely so. Jenny's mother died suddenly five years ago."

"What happened?"

"She had a heart attack. Her doctor would not believe her chest pain was caused by heart disease. She seemed too young. No one else in her family had ever had heart disease. The doctor decided to take out her gall bladder in order to relieve her pain. Her gall bladder was completely normal. During the postoperative period, her heart stopped beating. They made a desperate atttempt to save her. It was quite a scene. But she died."

The new information startled me. Jeb and Tina had been angry about conditions most people endure in silence, yet they had silently borne the burden of a family teetering on its pins. Jeb had been the stalwart support, the sensible head, the planner. Until he developed cancer, he had been the least dispensable.

"Your family has been torn apart by illness."

"It's just one of those things," Jeb said. "If you know enough about any family, they all have their tragedies. But you know, one thing sticks in my craw."

"What's that?"

"Dr. Carver saw my mother eight months ago. He has never asked me how she was doing. When he saw me this morning, he acted like he didn't even notice she had died."

"Perhaps he didn't know about it."

"He *should* have. He was one of her doctors."

"I'm sorry to have to talk to you about your cancer on the day your mother died. I guess you need some time to deal with your feelings," I said.

"Not at all," Jeb answered. "We knew mother was going to die for months. She had no energy. She would not eat. She sat and stared at the wall. At least she died in her sleep while Jenny was at school."

"This way we didn't have to tell Mom about Jeb," Tina added. "We told her Jeb was seriously ill and might lose his hair, but we did not tell her he was going to die. We let her hope."

"It's good to hope," I said.

They looked at me grimly.

"How can you say that when you know how bad things are for me?" Jeb asked.

"A decade ago I had a patient with the same kind of lung cancer you have. Only his spread to his brain. By all odds he should have died in one year, but he lived for nine. I don't think it ever hurts to have hope."

Hope is the one candle left fluttering in the darkness when all the others have been snuffed out. Caught in the presumption that more life is better, I long for any chance that my patients will outlive my expectations. I am especially gratified when they do.

A few weeks later, Dr. Carver called me. His voice trembled as he told me about Jeb.

"The cancer is growing," he said. "He hasn't much time left. I can't stay angry with these people. They've suffered too much."

For the next month, Jeb went for radiation therapy, meanwhile continuing to have fluid removed from his chest with a needle every week or two. Despite shortness of breath, progressive weakness, and daily trips to one or two doctors' offices, he continued to work.

When the radiation therapy was completed, Jeb switched from Dr. Carver to Dr. Sutton, a second pulmonary specialist.

"It's nothing personal," he told me. "I have great professional regard for Dr. Carver. I just don't like the way his office operates."

"We bent over backwards to please those people," Dr. Carver told me when I asked him about the switch. "All we got in return was criticism and a lack of cooperation. I don't bear them any malice, but our whole staff had grown tired of their aggressive behavior."

The spiral of anger had not ended. Within a month Jeb switched pulmonary specialists again. He had fired four doctors in six months. Moreover, each of the doctors he had fired had tried to appease him. I began to wonder whether Jeb would ever find relief.

"I liked Dr. Sutton's billing procedures better," Jeb said, "but he insisted that I have the fluid removed in the emergency room. I hated the emergency room. No one seemed to know what they were doing. I had to wait more than two hours for Dr. Sutton. No one could reach him. Tina was upset. I'm going to Dr. Mack now." Dr. Mack was kind to Jeb and Tina. He listened to Jeb's story from the start, discovering details I had missed. Something of a curmudgeon himself, he shared some of their rage. He soon became a trusted ally.

Jeb continued to work, although he did not feel better.

"I can't walk more than ten steps without stopping to rest," he told me.

"And yet you go to work?" I asked.

"That's right," he said. "I take the subway downtown. The stop is two blocks from my office. I can walk it in twenty minutes. My heart races, I pant for breath, I stop at every store window, but I make it. I put in half a day. Then I come home again."

"Are you able to perform well?" I asked.

"I'm slow, but I get the job done. At half speed I'm still above average for the civil service."

We both laughed.

"Do you think it's harmful?"

"No. But I think you will not be able to do it much longer. It sounds like your weakness will keep you home in bad weather. Winter's almost here. What do you plan to do if it snows?"

"I want to work another two and a half years so that my wife will get a pension. I try not to think about snow."

"Do you think that's a realistic goal?"

He nodded.

"I admire you, Jeb," I said.

Two weeks later, I was called to see Jeb at the hospital. He had been admitted with shortness of breath late the previous evening. By early morning his pulse had slowed, his blood pressure had dropped, and he had lost consciousness.

"I don't think he has long to live," I told the nurse. "I'll be right over."

By the time I reached the hospital, he had died.

"It wasn't supposed to happen like this!" Tina screamed. "The doctor last night told me he would be better this morning."

"I think he said that he *hoped* he would be better this morning. Something must have happened."

"What are you going to put on the death certificate?"

"Lung cancer."

"I know he had lung cancer, but he seemed to deteriorate suddenly as if something else were wrong with him."

I suggested several possibilities.

"I didn't have a chance to say good-bye," she said. "We had talked about it. Jeb had all but given up. We arranged the funeral together, picked out a plot, bought a stone. We even joked some time ago about being buried in the same grave with a trapdoor between the caskets. "Your place or mine?" he used to say. And I would say, "It all depends on who's on top." No one ever knew the kind of love we had. I will miss him forever."

Her eyes were clear. Her voice was steady. We talked about the events that led to Jeb's death.

"I know you always thought of me as hot-tempered and disagreeable," she said. "But all I wanted was what was best for Jeb."

"It showed, Tina," I said. "He was lucky to have you."

Given a taste of life's outer limits, some of us learn to appreciate the importance of human relationships and the insignificance of our anger. We learn to accept our families without imposing conditions on our love. We experience pure joy in an embrace. For the first time in our lives, it seems, we understand our relationship to God and our fellow human beings.

Sometimes, cancer helps to soothe angry feelings. Ethel had spent years living with anger, but her malignancy helped her to grow out of it.

I did not meet Ethel until her breast cancer had metastasized. She lived in a distant city and received most of her medical care near her home. Her breast cancer had been diagnosed six years earlier, just after her fifty-eighth birthday. A surgeon in my community had removed it and she had done well until she developed back pain. A bone scan had transformed Ethel from a woman who could contemplate decades of future life into a cancer patient who had but a few years remaining.

Unlike Jeb and Tina, Ethel did not look angry. She was rotund, slightly on the flabby side. She peeped at the world through narrowed eyes lodged in the recesses of a rounded face. No frown marks creased her brow. When she spoke, gentle tones and carefully chosen words were all she used. She did not gesture. Her anger lay buried, hidden by the slow pace of her speech. She seethed, but she seethed quietly. Gradually I learned to hear her anger.

"Shouldn't someone have done something to prevent this cancer from coming back?" she asked.

Her breast cancer surgery dated from the years when many women did not receive adjuvant therapy. Her surgeon had told her that he got it all. His sane advice, appropriate for the time, had become obsolete within a span of several years, but it had been too late for Ethel.

"With breast cancer we have more questions than answers. We rarely agree," I said. I described the consensus process by which American oncologists have tried to air their differences in a public forum. "With each new crop of large-scale studies on cancer, we come to new conclusions. Our aim is always the same: to do our best to cure as many women as we can. As a result, our advice changes often."

"But why didn't the doctor go over the possibilities?" she asked.

"I don't know."

"Didn't I have a right to choose which risks I wanted to take?" she asked.

"Of course. I encourage people to review their options with their doctors. The decisions affect their lives."

"I thought so," she said.

"You sound annoyed," I suggested.

"I wasn't given a choice," she said.

As the months passed, Ethel and I were pleased that the pain in her bones abated under the influence of a mild hormonal treatment. The cancer did not appear elsewhere. She had no symptoms of cancer, and yet she was still angry. I asked if she was annoyed about traveling three hours to my office. But she protested that she did not want an oncologist closer to home. She liked me. Yet every visit included mention of some detail of my behavior that "made her angry."

She was angry because I had failed to give her a report of her laboratory tests when she left the office. After that, I made copies of the data for her. She was angry because I had forgotten to write a letter to her physician each time she came. I made it my business to write more often. She was angry about our billing procedures. I arranged for her to have a conference with my billing office. She was angry because I had not told her about one of the side effects of the medication. I explained to her that the so-called side effect was quite rare.

Each time she expressed anger, I gave her additional time to talk. Each time I resolved the conflict. Yet with each new visit, she was angry again.

After many visits, with flushed face and tears in her eyes, she told me, "I have a confession to make."

From the tone of her voice, I guessed she was about to tell me she had done something truly outrageous, something worthy of publication in a supermarket tabloid. I settled back in my chair with my best listening expression.

"My son is an alcoholic," she said.

I tried to remain impassive, but it was difficult to conceal my disappointment. The problem was so ordinary. I wondered why, in the modern era, acknowledging the presence of an alcoholic in the family caused such agonies of guilt that confessing it to a doctor should be a momentous issue. Hundreds of people have told me about alcoholism in their spouses, parents, and offspring with much less guilt than Ethel had. Indeed, people have told me about rape, incest, and murder with less emotion than Ethel seemed to feel as she told me about her trials with her son. I wondered why.

"I have read that alcoholism is hereditary," she said. "But neither his father nor I are alcoholics. We have a drink once or twice a week. Never more."

"It can run in families, but there are many exceptions. In any case, it's not your fault."

"But I tried to be a good parent. I must have failed."

"Why do you say that?"

"He has always been a disappointment. He's gone from one failure to the next. First with his education, then with his efforts at earning a living. He had the best schools but he refused to study. We loaned him money to get started in business, not once but several times. What do we get in return? A drunk. He's been arrested several times. It's a small town. I feel mortified when he calls me from the jail."

"It must be painful," I said.

"But he's not stupid. He admits that he's an alcoholic. He always promises to be better. I try to believe him, but in my heart I know he's lying. He betrays me every time."

"Betrays *you*?" I asked.

She looked at me sharply, stunned.

"Do you think he wants to be an alcoholic, to fail at everything he tries, to be hauled off to jail, and to have to face your obvious disappointment? It bothers me, and I'm not even your son." And then, by luck rather than by wit, I managed to keep silent long enough for her to tell me, in a rush, all the misery that was in her heart. For the next half hour we both forgot that my job was to treat her cancer.

She returned three months later, this time with smiles. She gave me a hug before she sat down.

"What's that for?" I asked.

"Your caring," she said.

Two years have passed since that conversation. We've been together many times, always grateful for the chance to exchange news, even when it isn't good.

In the meantime, her husband died. She had been quite dependent on him, but she weathered widowhood without collapsing from the strain. Her breast cancer still has not come back.

We've talked about many things. Sometimes we talk about her son's slow recovery. Sometimes we talk about Ethel's recovery. She's learned to stop "expecting" things from him. She knows alcoholism is his disease, not hers.

"Learn to like yourself," she said one day when we were together. "Don't let your frustrations feed your anger. It doesn't make you happier. Think of your disappointments as projects, and work on them. Don't bolster your misery by dwelling on failures, yours or other people's. Take heart in your successes. Ask what you can do better. Then do it."

7
DENIAL

"You know how some people are," Dr. Starch told me when he asked me to care for Toby. "Denial prevents them from recognizing the seriousness of their illness."

Denial, a word which comes a bit too easily to doctors' tongues, is a term used to define a mental state in which *other* people ignore the obvious. We are sometimes tempted to accuse our patients of *ignoring* what we thought they should have seen. We use the term *denial* to explain behavior that does not make sense to us. But denial, like beauty, is in the eye of the beholder.

"*Some people,*" Dr. Starch had said. He seemed to imply that denial affected the mentally obtuse. Yet denial is ubiquitous, affecting people of all levels of intelligence. It is a rare individual who has never "ignored" something "obvious" to everyone else.

Toby did not discuss the six months that elapsed between his first symptom and the diagnosis of his cancer. He seemed disposed to focus his attention on coping with the present and planning for the future. He had no stomach for retrospection.

Ginny, initially outraged at Dr. Starch's "failure" to diagnose her husband's cancer, later told me she was grateful her husband's diagnosis had been delayed for six months. It had spared him what would surely have been constant worry about an incurable disease that would not have been easier to manage if we had known about it sooner. Indeed, we all believed an earlier diagnosis *would not have helped Toby.*

Paradoxically, denial is a necessary refuge for the curious. The ancient Hebrews, who encouraged learning, realized the pain of too much knowledge. They believed God, in His kindness, only revealed what was good for humans to know. They believed it was wicked to seek to know "the hidden things." Greek philosophers and modern scientists dared to peel away the covers, but they didn't make it easy for us. With knowledge of painful, inescapable conditions comes a wrenching rearrangement of our internal order. Awareness of new information forces us to grapple with chilling possibilities. Small wonder many of us cloak ourselves in denial, a temporary comfort, but a comfort just the same. If denial gave Toby six months of comfort, it was more effective for his kind of lung cancer than standard chemotherapy.

Toby could recognize and acknowledge his anxiety. He could identify his anger. He could admit he felt elation and depression, comfort and distress. But he never recognized denial in himself. When I visited Toby, despite his questions, his interest, and his anxiety, I often felt as if he had separated himself from his cancer. He acted as if his death might not happen because he was not ready for it.

Toby had a tendency to ignore unpleasant, frightening things when he discussed his illness with me. The rigidity of his body and his frightened stare made me aware of a sense of caution in myself, a reluctance to volunteer information which might prove threatening.

When Ginny talked about Toby, she stressed his realistic attitude, his awareness of his cancer, his willingness to talk about it. Others confirmed her opinion. Perhaps his behavior when he was with me was a necessary shield against the power of my authority. Perhaps his simplistic attitude in my presence prevented him from hearing statements that might have been unbearably frightening.

Denial, like beauty, is in the eye of the beholder.

Denial is not a feeling but a way of avoiding uncomfortable feelings. Rather than suffer the pain of confrontation, denial shuts painful reality out of conscious awareness. Shielded by denial, the stimuli for anxiety and anger diminish; the mind can attempt more tranquil thoughts.

Because we each see reality from a unique point of view, denial, of necessity, is different for each of us. Comedians make use of our contrasting perceptions of reality. As J. B. Cabell said, "The optimist proclaims that we live in the best of all possible worlds, and the pessimist fears this is true." We chuckle at the joke about the fellow who asked a man with a banana in his ear why it was there. The man replied, "I'm sorry, I can't hear you. I have a banana in my ear." Who was farther out of touch, the man with the banana in his ear or the man who would listen seriously to his explanation for putting it there?

Denial lends humor to the joke about a psychiatrist and a man whose sister thought she was a chicken. When the psychiatrist asked the man how long his sister had harbored such an outlandish idea the man replied, "All her life. We probably should have done something about it sooner but we needed the eggs."

We have all lived through rotten, unacceptable situations, ignoring the severity of the problem until one day when we took account of the situation. Suddenly we felt as startled as if we had been in a darkened room and someone had opened the curtains, flooding the room with sunlight. In looking back we wonder how any sane person could have endured such an extreme situation without noticing it, how we could ever have believed that the "chicken" was actually laying eggs.

A diagnosis of cancer is one of those experiences that suddenly calls us to account. As it strips away our privacy, it tears at our denial, too. Not content to stop with our clothes, radiologists peer within each body segment; gastroenterologists, armed with fiber optics, spy through our orifices; surgeons explore our abdomens; pathologists analyze our blood and slice and serve our tissues under glass; internists tell us what is wrong with our bodies; and psychiatrists ask us how the information affects us.

But it does not stop there. For when we return home, the telephone begins to ring. Friends, relatives, know-it-alls, long-lost contacts, someone who knows a little medicine, and a neighbor we've scarcely met join in the circus. Armed with questions, articles, home-remedy books, and too many anecdotes to mention, they too invade. While the people in the hospital may have shown some delicacy, one of our visitors is certain to tell us we should have known something everyone else had missed. And like the emperor wearing invisible clothes, we turn to listen to the uninhibited speaker who, fearless of the consequences of telling the truth, blurts it out in public. This childlike voice tells us our denial was foolish and leaves us naked and ashamed.

An oncology nurse, a close friend of mine, determined to be "open" about her breast cancer, was amazed at the barrage from her acquaintances. "They mean well," she said. "And some of them were awfully sweet. But there were so many of them, and they all wanted to know everything about me. I felt as stripped of my dignity as a Thanksgiving turkey after the meal."

No wonder we seek denial in an attempt to return to normalcy. In fact, people who can't protect themselves by denial can achieve some comfort by faking it.

Experience can change our view of reality. What we deny at one time may appear to be unquestioned verities at another: our perception does not necessarily improve with age, but it is likely to be altered. Driving well beyond the speed limit looks vastly different to my teenaged son than it does to his father. My increasing decrepitude on the ski slopes is much less obvious to me than it is to him.

When I see cartons of cigarettes these days, I see packaged death. Years ago, when I still smoked, I saw pleasure, relaxation, a chance to break the monotony. When people warned me of the hazards of smoking, I accused them of exaggerating. The moment of my epiphany arrived when I was serving as an intern. I was responsible for three men who were victims of nicotine addiction. All had cigarette-induced disease. One had a nearly fatal heart attack at the age of thirty-eight. The second had lung cancer. And the third, a man I was examining when the revelation occurred, had developed cancer of the larynx. To rid the third man of his cancer, a surgeon had removed his larynx. He was forced to breathe through a hole in the bottom of his neck, a permanent tracheostomy. At the moment I arrived on the ward, the man was smoking a king-sized cigarette through his tracheostomy. Cigarettes had caused irreversible damage to his body, yet he was still smoking.*

My wall of denial crumbled. As I peered into the blackened hole at the base of his neck, I saw myself slipping painfully into a well of self-destruction. I threw out a package of nineteen cigarettes and never purchased another one.

Although I could not cure these men, witnessing the harmful effects of smoking cured me. I have never smoked since. And I have never clearly understood my denial. Indeed, before I started to smoke, I had been keenly aware of the risks. Before I saw the three men on the ward, I had known of many diseases caused by smoking. I knew that smoke sucked through the mouth enters the lungs. I had seen the blackened lungs of smokers removed at autopsy. I knew about the quart of tar that accumulates in the lung tissues during the many "pack-years" of a smoker's life. Facts did not alter my denial. The physical experience of watching the smoke disappear into the pink hole in my patient's neck had more impact than hours of teaching and hectoring.

Because of my own experience, I do not condemn denial in others. I saw addiction rather than moral weakness when counseling a woman who had not stopped smoking when her father developing lung cancer. I saw fear, not stupidity, in a biochemist who had a lump the size of a grapefruit in one of his testes but waited a year to seek medical attention. I did not challenge the explanations of the married(!) woman who had an oozing mass

*_Dead Again_, a recently released film, shows a supporting character smoking through a tracheostomy. Perhaps viewing this macabre sight may be therapeutic for smokers who need to witness such an event to be shaken from their addiction.

instead of a breast, who had clearly known about her problem for years, but who had never seen a physician. I know about denial. It is everywhere.

Denial of the symptoms of cancer is like denial of other threats to life. It makes it possible for us to act as if we were safe from the hazards that surround us. Flashing lights warn drivers to slow for highway construction. How many do? The American Cancer Society vigorously promotes mammograms as a means of saving lives, but how many heed its call? The same *normal* behavior that makes it possible for us to avoid following sensible advice when we are well makes it possible, when we are ill, to ignore internal changes, the admonitions of friends and family, and all the education life has given us.

The denial associated with malignancy often develops slowly, in parallel with the growth of cancer cells. People accommodate to the presence of cancer, ignoring symptoms or giving them another explanation. An event occurs. Someone makes them see a doctor. Suddenly, they see what was previously invisible. They are shocked at their "stupidity." The doctors may have missed the early signs of cancer, too. Despite years of experience, even a seasoned professional can push away unpleasant facts.

With denial stripped away, shock may turn to anger. Anger at themselves for "ignoring" the truth. Anger at their doctors for supporting their ignorance instead of forcing them to seek facts. Indeed, their physicians may be angry at themselves.

Doctors use technology to overcome denial. Scrupulous data collection can help people confront medical facts. Modern instruments help physicians avoid some of the errors of their predecessors. But denial continues to thrive.

To be certain, we have learned to eschew the practices of eighteenth-century physicians who drained pints of blood from the sick with the staunch conviction that it was good for them.* We are appalled by the physicians who lethally exsanguinated George

*Some would argue that the daily rites of the hospital phlebotomists are the evolutionary offspring of the leeches and lances of the eighteenth century.

Washington in the conviction that he "needed" it for his quinsy throat. We ridicule the nineteenth-century surgeons who took delight in the purulent reactions of infected wounds. Why couldn't they see how they were killing their patients?

But denial is still alive and well. Even now, we continue to treat illnesses with unproven remedies or remedies proven ineffective. We ignore correctable problems in people who feel well, even when we know the high price of delay. We avoid advising people about smoking, alcohol, and seat belts. We act as if these problems are not important even though statistics tells us otherwise.

But perhaps the most severe form of denial in the modern era is the inability to see the harm we doctors cause by creating invisible problems like mental suffering. Whether we are defensive or offensive, arrogant or elegant, abrupt or windy, we share a trait which people with serious problems like cancer have come to loathe. We act as if the mental suffering produced by too much medical information, technical language, refusal to answer questions, controlling behavior, impatience, confusing directions, lengthy delays, excessive fees, failure to return telephone calls, inaccessibility, delegation of tasks which should be done by physicians, and inadequate preparation of patients for side-effects and complications were not our responsibility. Whose is it, then? Only when we doctors feel as much concern for the human anguish we create as we do for blood loss or infected wounds will this form of denial begin to erode.

Not far removed from physician denial of mental anguish is our ability to ignore or undertreat pain. Our chart notes do not reflect the way people feel because our patients often do not discuss such sensitive topics as freely as objective issues, but hearing well means listening to such complaints, even if it requires extra time and much prompting. Physician neglect of these issues is rampant denial of a central tenet of medicine: To cure sometimes, to comfort always. Physicians who don't agree should try being sick for a while.

Besides being universal and insidious, denial is a somewhat fuzzy process. At the periphery of denial lie ignorance, inattention, and distraction. No one can be certain when the borders are located.

A case in point: Marvin was a sixty-four-year-old engineer who was referred to me because of anemia. He had been seriously ill. To be sure, he had undergone surgery for gallstones and appendicitis. Until the mid twentieth century, such surgery would have entailed a substantial risk of death. But now, with good anesthesia, with fiber optics and microsurgical techniques, with effective antibiotics and good postoperative care, such surgery rarely causes more than a brief disturbance in the pace of life. In any case, from Marvin's point of view, he had been a healthy man. As a consequence, he had not seen a physician in years.

One day Marvin had a severe pain in his chest. A doctor gave Marvin an anti-inflammatory agent, based on the suspicion that the pain arose from the rib joints. She encouraged Marvin to have a physical examination. During the physical examination, both doctor and patient decided Marvin's chest pain was related to exertion. Coronary artery disease was suspected. Indeed, all of Marvin's family had suffered from atherosclerosis, and several among his parents' generation had died from it. A stress test was ordered. Marvin's doctor included a hemoglobin among the two dozen laboratory tests which she ordered in preparation for the stress test. As a result, she discovered a mild anemia, possibly a result of the anti-inflammatory drug. In any case, the doctor chose to evaluate the chest pain because of the possibility of an impending heart attack.

Because his stress test showed clear signs of angina, Marvin consulted a cardiologist. Soon afterwards, he had an angiogram that showed major blockage of five coronary blood vessels. The cardiologist advised Marvin to have surgery at once. During coronary artery bypass grafting, Marvin received four units of blood as a matter of routine. He left the hospital after an uneventful stay. But two days later, he returned with chest pain and a fever. His doctor suspected a complication of surgery and treated him accordingly. Again he received an anti-inflammatory drug. Marvin's anemia was worse. His doctor spoke with the cardiologist, who told him most patients are anemic after bypass surgery. Marvin received another transfusion. His temperature returned to normal, and he was discharged.

A week after the second discharge, he returned with acute kidney failure. The kidney failure puzzled Marvin's doctors, but they suspected that the anti-inflammatory agent caused it. They stopped the medication, and the kidney failure improved, but Marvin was still anemic. His doctor ordered laboratory tests to diagnose the anemia. All were normal. The cardiologist suggested Marvin's slow recovery from the anemia might have been due to the kidney failure. The doctor ordered another transfusion.

A month later, Marvin required yet another transfusion. Marvin had six conscientious internists by then. All of them had elicited the same information. The cause of the anemia was still undetermined. His family doctor became concerned. She suggested Marvin see me for a hematology consultation.

During the two months following his heart surgery, Marvin had not felt well. He was constantly tired. He ached. He had no energy. But these nonspecific symptoms were all easily explained by problems he had encountered after the surgery.

After listening to his story and examining all of the data he brought with him, I told Marvin I thought it unlikely we would find another explanation for the anemia easily. Nevertheless, I decided I would examine his bone marrow, just to be certain it looked normal.

I obtained the bone marrow specimen at four o'clock on a Friday. I stained a portion of it quickly. While Marvin and his wife waited in my office, I examined it under the microscope. Normal bone marrow contains a wide variety of cells, but Marvin's was monotonous. Abnormal, malignant-looking plasma cells crowded together like swarms of wasps. Few normal cells could be seen. A medical student could have made a diagnosis of myeloma.

Within an hour of meeting Marvin for the first time, I had made a diagnosis that had eluded experienced physicians for months. Until I made my discovery, sick as he had been, his doctors had explained every symptom of myeloma with another diagnosis. In an instant, their "denial" of the true cause of Marvin's chest pain (cracked ribs), anemia (bone marrow replacement), and kidney failure (myeloma protein) had been destroyed. A single diagnostic test had changed Marvin's illnesses from survivable to fatal. At five o'clock on a Friday, it became my task to announce the change to a pair of strangers.

My explanation would have to convince them that a sliver of bone marrow, flattened between two tiny pieces of glass carried more diagnostic authority than his physicians had accumulated in three months of close observation. My opinion would take precedence over the advice his other doctors had given him. In essence, I would be opening Marvin's eyes to a form of medical denial. His doctors had thought they had explained Marvin's anemia, but they were wrong. Despite their copious tests, the error of their conclusions were as far from the truth as that of the young man with the enormous cancer in his testis who thought he had a bruise. Or the emperor who paraded through the streets in the buff.

Marvin and his doctors had taken each of his problems seriously. They gathered data, documented their diagnoses with appropriate tests. Their data explained the facts. His chest pain *could* have been explained by heart disease. His stress test *was* abnormal. His angiogram *did* show narrowed coronary arteries. The anti-inflammatory medication *could* have caused the anemia. The explanations accounted for Marvin's problems, but they were wrong.

Years of practicing medicine have made the patterns of my denial clearer to me. I am more likely to overlook certain symptoms. I must be particularly vigilant about fatigue, for example, because it is a common complaint, rarely related to a specific diagnosis. But on occasion it is the only symptom of a severe illness. Although it does not usually augur serious disease, I must avoid the assumption that it never does.

Marvin's problem underlines the inherent fallibility of medicine. Physicians can overcome denial because of their determination to improve their understanding of symptoms.*

Is constant vigilance and awareness of the hazards of denial enough to protect physicians from missing "reality" when confronted with clear evidence? The public expects it of us. Litigious patients sue us when we fail. And I suspect such errors happen regularly to most physicians. Oversights occur even in academic centers, justifiably proud of their thorough evaluations, abundantly staffed with doctors whose goal is to miss nothing remotely relevant.

A patient was transferred to my care by a prestigious institution. Her symptoms were as confusing to her doctors as they were to her. A week before, well-trained doctors had evaluated her without success. Two days following the transfer, by performing a CAT scan of her head, I was able to explain her symptoms. A test which any doctor could have ordered solved a problem that had eluded other physicians for weeks.

In defining denial, we are forced to recognize human limitations. Some patients expect almost magical perfection from physicians. They act as if even momentary delays in diagnosis were egregious errors. Some physicians expect perfection from themselves. They suffer paroxysms of guilt about oversights so small that they are difficult to describe.

An expectation of human perfection is itself an exquisite form of denial.

A woman—I'll call her Ruby—complained to her rheumatologist about her hip. She had walked into his office, using her walker. Her body was contorted by severe arthritis, and she had often

*Sophisticated readers may wonder whether Marvin's physicians missed the tip-off of an elevated globulin on the chemistry profile. Unfortunately, Marvin's myeloma did not secrete whole immunoglobulins. He had hypogammaglobulinemia with "light-chain" proteinuria.

complained of pain in many joints, especially her hips. On examination, she looked much as she had on previous visits. The doctor changed Ruby's pain medication but did not take an X-ray because he "knew it would show severe arthritis." Shortly afterward, I admitted her to the hospital because she was confused and short of breath. She had pain in her right hip as well as other problems. Aided by several consultants, I treated her confusion and her breathing problem; then, towards the *end* of her hospital stay and for vague reasons which I cannot justify, I ordered an X-ray of her hip. To my surprise, the X-ray showed a fracture that was probably three weeks old and previously unrecognized by me, a rheumatologist, and three consultants. Indeed, to add to the irony, simplemindedness, rather than mental subtlety, had led me to the diagnosis. If I had thought more deeply about her rheumatoid arthritis, I probably would not have ordered the X-ray, because I would have been "certain" that it would not add any information. As it was, her persistent complaint of pain and her relative immobility bothered me enough to do what any nonphysician would have suggested immediately. Denial hovers like a dense cloud ready to befog people who know too much. To overcome denial, we must harken to unlikely and, sometimes, unwelcome voices. Sometimes innocence, rather than experience, provides the clearest view.

I can only guess about Toby's use of denial. I did not meet him until more than half a year after the onset of his symptoms. I could not assess his reaction. I do not know whether Toby had avoided seeking help because he "knew too much" or whether, trusting his physicians, he was content to live with his symptoms because he "did not know enough" to recognize that something serious was happening to him.

My uncertainty about Toby is similar to my feelings about the experienced doctors who came to believable but incorrect conclusions about Marvin. All of the doctors knew about myeloma. They all knew that it caused anemia, bone pain, kidney failure, weakness, and fatigue. Any one of them could have suspected the diagnosis. But they operated on false assumptions, just as Toby did. And just as Marvin's narrowed coronary arteries *could have* accounted for his chest pain but didn't, bronchitis *could have* caused Toby's cough but didn't.

Whenever I am tempted to diagnose denial, I feel as if the onus were on me to define reality. The diagnosis of denial is inappropriate if my patient lacked the intellectual power to perceive that reality. An accurate diagnosis of denial is a philosopher's dream, a clinician's nightmare.

A recent experience serves as an example of the confusion of reality in the world of medicine. I was asked to see an eighty-one-year-old woman who was being cared for by two other doctors. One of them had written a note in her chart: "Doing well post-operatively but moderately confused. She insists that she is going to have a CAT scan tomorrow." The confusion was on the part of the physician. Her other doctor *had* ordered a CAT scan. Indeed the woman had the permission slip for the procedure in her hand when I visited her. In a crackling voice she remarked to me that she was old but not dumb.

Toby was neither old nor dumb. The reality of his illness plagued him because it kept him from doing what he most loved: jogging. I was not there to witness his explanation of the decline, the reactions of his friends and relatives to the unusually severe distress his "bronchitis" caused him. Accordingly, I cannot judge the degree to which denial delayed his return to medical care as his stamina underwent a severe, unexpected decline.

I did see something in Toby later, a quality that might serve as a warning to others who are at risk of avoiding medical care because of denial. Toby appeared to feel uncomfortable whenever we discussed his disease. Although he spent his professional life dealing with facts and information, although he was organized, bright, disciplined, and mature, whenever I tried to discuss his cancer, his level of tolerance proved marginal. With sighs, digressions, and body language he bid me stop. After I stopped, he did not urge me to resume.

He never pumped me with questions, made long lists of information, scrutinized his X-rays, debated the advantages and disadvantages of various treatments. Rather, he approached key issues, palpably anxious about my answers, prepared to limit my responses. When, in deference to his wishes, I gave only the briefest answers, he would smile and say, "You seem to know me pretty well."

What has all that to do with denial?

People who want to avoid hearing facts send me a message: Your facts are painful. My intelligence is too keen to ignore them. My psyche is too fragile to cope with them.

No concern is more properly a part of the doctor–patient relationship than an implied contract about the style, quantity, and quality of the information that will be shared both ways. To the extent that denial affects us all, it may play a part in the contracts doctors and patients make with each other. But it's a part I can never measure, only guess about. Asking people about the severity of their denial makes as much sense as asking them if they are asleep.

A patient named Laura gave a lucid description of the delicate nature of the transmission of information. She told me she had sought the opinion of a radiation therapist. In the course of their discussion, the therapist calmly informed Laura that she had only a 35 percent chance of being cured by the treatment I had given her. Laura had not asked the therapist what her chances were or whether she would be cured. Furthermore, she did not want to know. Numbers of that sort frightened her. To make matters worse, Laura suffered from chronic depression. "Bad news" tended to make her depression worse. She interpreted the radiation therapist's prognosis as bad news. After several miserable weeks, she came to me for reassurance.

"Tell me the facts if they're good," she said. "Otherwise, I just don't want to know."

The facts, as it turned out, were considerably better than the radiation therapist had stated. Laura wished to limit the number of factual conversations about her cancer. The radiation therapist believed Laura's denial was bad for her. Who was entitled to decide?

Laura participated in the medical decisions at a level that was comfortable for her. She only wanted answers to the questions she asked. She saw no benefit from the additional emotional pain of being given frightening statistics.

People react to numbers differently. Some are reassured by being told they have a 35 percent chance of survival, others are terrified by it.

When Toby coughed up blood, he suspected serious illness and sought medical advice. He followed the doctor's orders carefully. Despite discomfort, expense, and anxiety about the outcome, Toby underwent all the tests his doctor ordered. Dr. Starch told him that he did not have cancer. At least, that's what Toby heard. Neither Dr. Starch nor Toby thought that denial was a factor in their conversations.

Six months later, the issue of denial created anger. Dr. Starch thought that denial had prevented Toby from seeking treatment earlier; Toby thought Dr. Starch should have warned him what might happen.

Perhaps few subjects in medicine excite more anger than a "delay" in diagnosis. When months or years intervene between the first visit with a complaint and the diagnosis of malignancy, some patients accuse their doctors of negligence. But even careful doctors delay making diagnoses. Early cancers can be extremely subtle.

Denial can sometimes be overcome by insisting that all parties listen to each other. Marvin and Toby and their wives, for example, had noticed symptoms that did not completely fit the diagnoses they had been given. More time spent talking in their doctors' offices might have led to a clearer understanding about what was wrong. Instead of encouraging conversation, however, we often abbreviate it in the interest of performing objective tests. Unfortunately, objective tests can be misleading. Subjective observations, properly interpreted, remain our most sensitive instruments in the diagnosis of most medical problems.

A fund of knowledge is not a safeguard against denial. Physicians with cancer commonly exhibit severe denial. One doctor, who had noticed blood in his stools for more than a year before his colon cancer was diagnosed, told his doctor that he believed the blood had been caused by hemorrhoids. He had never had a rectal examination. A second physician had blood in his urine for nearly as long before a bladder cancer was found.

"I knew that blood in the urine may be the only symptom of a bladder cancer," he told his urologist. "But I am a jogger. I thought jogging was causing the blood." Jogging occasionally causes red urine, but no nonphysician would have dared to risk his life on such an assumption. As every doctor learns in his training, blood in the urine is a sign of cancer until proven otherwise.

Not only is intelligence no safeguard against denial, a fund of medical information may increase denial. An alarming number of physicians continue to smoke. One might guess that such physicians were less exposed to patients who had suffered from the hazardous consequences of the addiction, but the opposite is the case. The smokers I know include pulmonary specialists, thoracic surgeons, cardiologists, and oncologists, all of whom have seen a greater-than-average share of cigarette-induced disease and death. They have experienced the grief at close range. Many of them make their patients stop smoking but continue to smoke themselves. I knew two chest surgeons who were smokers. Both of them had operated on hundreds of patients with lung cancer before dying of the disease themselves. A medical oncologist in our community smoked two packs a day. He died suddenly of a heart attack during his morning shower. Denial is not due to a lack of intelligence, experience, or knowledge.

Denial does not affect people because they fail to care but rather because they care too much. I was made aware of my own susceptibility to denial when one of my children began to lose weight.

From the time we brought our first baby home, I have always had a heightened awareness of the diseases that can affect children. My imagination blossomed with frightening possibilities. A fever made me think of bacterial sepsis, even though it was probably due to a virus. A headache suggested fatal meningitis, even though it disappeared in a few hours. Although I worried about unlikely possibilities, I never mentioned my fears to anyone. Instead, I wore the physician's look of confidence. My appearance of calm enabled my family to accept their illnesses without undue concern. For my first nineteen years as a parent, I don't believe I ever ignored a serious problem or failed to bring my children to prompt medical attention when they needed it. My daughter's weight loss was different.

It was subtle at first. Her pudgy face became elongated. Her rounded body assumed a more mature form. After all, I reasoned, she was ten years old. I expected changes to occur.

But I noticed a sad look about her eyes, as if she expected me to help her in some vague way. It was an expression I could not quite understand. I remember feeling something was wrong, but I was easily distracted. I was afraid she was going to die. The feelings disappeared in fractions of a second, eclipsed by other thoughts. My professional life consumed much of my time. We filled our leisure hours with exciting activities. We almost never took time to stop and think. And the child who had visibly lost weight, whose health was more important to me than my professional life or any of those leisure-time activities, did not enter my consciousness because I could not tolerate the thought that something terrible was happening to her.

In the midst of the weight loss, my wife and I took our daughter by train to New York City to see a Degas show at the Metropolitan Museum. Shortly before the trip, our daughter had sprained her ankle. She had been told to use crutches to allow it to heal.

Despite its reputation in some quarters, New York can be a remarkably friendly city. Everywhere we went, people were helpful to us. In the Empire State Building people cheerfully answered our questions. On the Madison Avenue bus an artist who had just landed a calendar contract gave us samples of her work. Other passengers helped us to wrap them. A friendly couple helped us find the right stop for the museum. The exhibit was everything we expected, and the three of us delighted in seeing every picture in it. Afterwards, we headed down to Rumpelmayer's for ice cream and a walk along Fifth Avenue.

Amidst all the excitement in New York, I could ignore a nagging concern that was easily chased from my consciousness. But given time to reflect on the train ride home, I suddenly became aware of what was worrying me. My daughter's face was *too* thin. Her cheeks were hollow and her eyes slightly sunken. I knew children do not normally lose weight. Because I am an oncologist, one, and only one, possibility occurred to me. But even as I thought of it, the pain of giving it serious consideration made it vanish.

For two weeks, which in retrospect seemed much longer, instead of taking action about something I suspected was quite serious, I continued to work, engage in family activities, and distract myself. I could not even bring myself to ask my wife to take my daughter to the pediatrician.

Then late one evening, my wife commented about our daughter's remarkable thirst.

"My God!" I said, sitting stark upright in bed. "She has diabetes. That explains everything!" And I nearly wept with a joy I found difficult to explain.

The following day, my wife took her to the pediatrician, stopping on the way to have a blood test performed. The doctor, whose youngest daughter has diabetes, thought it unlikely that our daughter had the same disease.

"We'll wait for the blood test results," he said. "But she can go to school."

Within an hour, we were told her blood sugar was six times normal. Diabetes was the only possible cause. As we whisked her off to the hospital, I struggled to avoid clutching to the fantastic belief that the diabetes would go away, that it was all a bad dream from which I would soon awake.

Two days later, my daughter helped banish my absurd longings.

"People have sent me balloons that say 'Get Well Soon!' " she said, "but I'm not going to get well, am I, Daddy?"

Fortunately, we were soon surrounded by competent physicians, nurses, social workers, nutritionists, a parent support group, the Juvenile Diabetes Foundation, and an enormously supportive family. We learned to live with the reality of diabetes on a daily basis. As for the future, distraction rather than denial helped us cope with what we could not predict. We knew what *might* happen, not what *would*, and we dealt with present problems rather than future imponderables. Friends sent us clippings of newspaper articles. The pediatrician encouraged us. A close colleague, a fellow oncologist, sent me a letter when he heard about my daughter. His twenty-two-year-old son had developed diabetes when he was six. The disease had not prevented him from growing into a strong, active adult. He had been a good student as well as an exercise enthusiast and was currently enrolled in medical school. Indeed, my colleague went on to say, people with diabetes could live nearly normal lives.

My friend's letter worked its charm on me. I looked at my daughter's diabetes with renewed optimism.

Incidently, my daughter seems less inclined to use denial as a defense than I do. In honor of my birthday, she wrote a little story:

THE LIFE OF A ROSE

A rose is born into a beautiful life. Everyone looks at the rose and admires it. It is seen as very precious and quite sacred. The rose is placed in a beautiful vase for all to see.

When the flower begins to die, it is immediately moved and no longer respected. The rose loses its value and is forgotten, but that is wrong. The rose should not be discarded; it may not be beautiful any more, but it is still a rose and should always be loved and never mistreated.

I love you, Dad. Happy Birthday.

As I listen to horror stories about other doctors who "ignored" medical problems and didn't "seem to care" what was happening to their patients, I wonder how many of those doctors are victims of the same phenomenon that affected me. How many have learned to conceal their feelings in order to protect their patients from undue alarm? How many have avoided searching for unlikely but life-threatening causes of symptoms in order to spare their patients anguish and unnecessary expense? How many have shielded their patients, not because they did not care about them, but because they cared too much? For no matter how many times I tell myself I am not the cause of my patients' illnesses, I always feel a heavy load when a test I have performed helps establish a diagnosis of a fatal illness.

Toby did not cease to use denial after the diagnosis was made. In contrast to people who speak of their cancers in realistic terms and press for increased knowledge about their progression, Toby hesitated to be blunt with me about it. He talked about remote possibilities as if they would surely happen. He reminded me of a Green Beret who was told that only one member of his squad was likely to survive a proposed assault on an enemy position. He was confident he would survive.

185
DENIAL

I think many people like to identify denial—in others. We were amused by the antics of a cartoon character, Mr. Magoo, whose severe myopia caused him to misconstrue what was happening to him. We laughed uproariously as he coasted through scenes strewn with wild animals, powerful machines, dangerous weapons, and malevolent evildoers. In keeping with his elaborate misconceptions, he remained unscathed despite the constant risk of injury. Mr. Magoo made a state of denial seem better than a state of reality.

Caring for people with cancer has guided me to the kernel of truth at the core of the Magoo stories. Most of us embrace some form of denial most of the time; if not about ourselves, then about our families, neighborhoods, city streets, highways, country, economy, or world. We act as if we were in control when we are not. We continue planning as if our lives depended on the structure we give to our activities, yet we remain oblivious to destruction in our midst.

As I wrote these words, many Americans were acting as if they were unaffected by the ongoing crisis in the Balkans, Africa, and the Middle East, the corruption in the financial world, the devastation of our inner cities, the proliferation of dangerous drugs and weapons, the plight of the jobless and those without health insurance, the deficiencies in our educational system and industrial productivity, the destruction of our environment, and the national debt. We were more easily aroused by isolated episodes of violence than we were by issues that threaten to make the world uninhabitable. Denial is a popular pastime.

Someone explained this paradox to me. "Individual criminals can be punished. Those other problems are beyond our reach."

Perhaps. But as we pretend to work on "law and order" while we ignore more important problems, are we not behaving like Mr. Magoo, who concentrated on putting sugar in his tea while his house collapsed around him?

The scientific method has stripped away most of my denial. But I know medical tests can only guarantee health *within limits*. I have been examined by a competent doctor. He told me I was in good health. Every test he did was normal. I even had a flexible sigmoidoscopy and a barium enema to exclude polyps and colon cancer. But people with normal blood pressure can still have strokes and heart disease. People with normal blood sugars can develop diabetes. People with normal cholesterols can die of heart attacks. People even develop colon cancer after a normal sigmoidoscopy and barium enema.

Knowing *that*, I can feel secure because I do not expect perfection from medical technology or my doctor.

But with all the frightening possibilities a doctor has to think about, how do I avoid worrying about my health? I concentrate on the needs of other people and act as if nothing is going to happen to me. If there's a bit of denial involved, I figure it helps me endure.

8
INFORMATION

"When *I* use a word," Humpty Dumpty said, in a rather scornful tone, "it means just what I choose it to mean—neither more nor less."

"The question is," said Alice, "whether you *can* make words mean so many different things."*

"WITH ALL the tests he did, why didn't my doctor make a diagnosis sooner?" Toby asked me. "I had the same complaints six months ago."

"What do you mean?" I asked.

"You told me Dr. Starch was one of the best lung specialists you know. Why didn't he see my lung cancer?"

When Toby asked me questions like this, I did not analyze his motives. He wanted to understand the world of medical information in the same way that he understood the world of computers. I wanted to help him despite the complexity of the topic. For even though I study constantly, I barely understand medicine

*Lewis Carroll (Charles Lutwidge Dodgson), *Alice Through the Looking-Glass*.

myself. Why indeed must the human body be so frustrating and complicated when the questions we ask are relatively simple? Why do tests mislead and treatments fail when logic would have predicted otherwise?

"When doctors look for a small object, like an early cancer, deep inside your body, it is as if they were fumbling in the dark. We can miss cancers that are too small to see. Months later, when the cancer has enlarged and we know precisely where it is, we sometimes think we should have seen it earlier. Our vision improves remarkably when we stare into the past.

"X-rays never show cancers, Toby," I added.

"What do you mean by that? Of course they do! Why bother with X-rays if they don't show cancers."

"I'm being cryptic, Toby," I said. "But I want to make a point. X-rays only show shadows, not diagnoses. People have learned to look at those shadows and recognize patterns. Some patterns suggest cancers with more certainty than others. Radiologists often read X-rays as 'consistent with cancer,' because other diseases could have a similar appearance. When we have proof of a diagnosis, the meaning of the patterns becomes clear. When the suspected diagnosis is cancer, the proof is obtained by biopsy. Dr. Starch did several biopies. None of them contained cancer cells. No cancer was found in the brushings he removed through the bronchoscope, either. Your symptom was a bloody cough. If cancer had caused the symptom, he expected to find some cancer cells in your airways. Finding none, Dr. Starch doubted that you had cancer. Bronchitis seemed to be a more likely cause of the bloody cough. Based on the evidence, Dr. Starch's reasoning was correct. But his diagnosis wasn't. Our reasoning is based on probabilities, not certainties."

"If I understand you right," Toby said, "You are telling me Dr. Starch did not know for certain *what* was wrong with me in July. *That's* what I misunderstood. When he said it was bronchitis, I thought he was certain of the diagnosis after he had done the bronchoscopy."

"A communication failure. Certainty is a medical rarity. If more people understood their doctors' doubts as well as their diagnoses, our communication would improve."

Brent was a twenty-eight-year-old man. When Brent was not working at his desk, he enjoyed vigorous exercise. He went for hikes. He rode a bicycle for thirty or forty miles at a stretch. He participated regularly in an organized volleyball league.

He came to see me because he had pain in his knee. I expected the usual signs of arthritis, but he had no stifness, redness, or swelling. Nevertheless, I suspected a "wear and tear" injury of his joint. Knee problems are common in young men who work at desks during the week and vigorously compete in the after hours. I told Brent to restrict his athletic activity, warm up carefully, quit at the first sign of pain, take aspirin, and come back in four weeks.

He stopped the hikes and the bicycle riding, warmed up before each activity, played less volleyball, and took the aspirin when he remembered. When he returned to the office he had less pain, but his knee continued to ache.

"I don't think it's in the joint," he said. He pointed to the end of his thighbone a few inches above the knee. "That's where it hurts the most."

"I still think it's wear and tear," I said. "It may not be arthritis. It's not typical."

I thought of shin splints, but those are *below* the knee, where Brent had no complaints. Athletes do not usually develop wear and tear pain a few inches above the knee, but I did not consider any other diagnoses at the time.

I sent him to an orthopedist for an examination and an X-ray. The X-ray was normal, and the orthopedist agreed with me. He increased the aspirin and the restrictions and told him to return if he did not improve. A month later, Brent called to say he was somewhat improved. I did not hear from him again for four months. Indeed, the next call came not from Brent himself but from another orthopedist.

"I do sports medicine," the second orthopedist said. "Brent was getting frustrated waiting out the knee injury. He came to me for advice about rehabilitation. I took another X-ray. To my surprise, I discovered cancer in his bone. That's why he hurts."

Fortunately, Brent had a giant cell tumor, a curable form of bone cancer. A surgeon was able to remove the tumor without sacrificing Brent's leg. After a few weeks, he had completed the treatment and was able to walk with crutches.

"Why didn't the first orthopedist find the cancer?" Brent asked me later. "It sounds like negligence."

"We looked at the X-ray again," I said. "Even when we knew a cancer was hidden in your thigh, we still couldn't see it."

"That's terrible," Brent said. "Your tests aren't worth much."

"Our tests aren't worthless, Brent. Modern technology helps us identify diseases with much more accuracy and much earlier than we ever could years ago. But it's still important to be humble about our accomplishments. No engineer has ever designed a diagnostic instrument as versatile and sensitive as the human body."

Pride in ourselves can blind us as effectively as denial. Because doctors have the same feelings as other humans, our pride can sometimes interfere with our handling of information. Because I believe we can all learn from understanding how it could interfere with good medical care, I have chosen to tell a story in which a doctor's pride nearly killed his patient.

The story does *not* involve an incompetent, ignorant, or immature physician or a patient who knew more about medicine than his physician. Rather, Dr. Prince had an international reputation as an authority in gastroenterology. Steve's knowledge of medicine was limited to a first-aid course.

Steve was thirty-three years old in 1978. As a Peace Corps officer he had been assigned to the Brazilian jungle. While in Brazil, he lost his appetite, became jaundiced, and developed a severe pain in his abdomen. In good health a few weeks earlier, he suddenly became gravely ill. His superiors sent him back to the United

States and arranged for him to be admitted to a teaching hospital.

The sudden onset of illness in the Brazilian jungle suggested a diagnosis of tropical infection to Dr. Prince, his attending physician. After preliminary evaluation, Dr. Prince told Steve he had hepatitis and not a tropical disease. In response to questions, Dr. Prince explained the implications of the disease to Steve and his wife, Liz, who was five months pregnant.

The next day, when Dr. Prince came by to see Steve, he was surprised to learn that the hepaititis tests were negative. Of more importance, a large mass had been discovered on the chest X-ray. The new finding made cancer highly likely.

Dr. Prince's face darkened when he spoke to Steve.

"This does not look good," he said.

Before Steve could ask him what he meant, Dr. Prince was gone. He did not describe the mass or the possible implications. He did not tell Steve what tests he planned to do. He did not ask Steve about his symptoms. He just left.

In the next few days, Steve was hustled through a series of tests. Afterwards, he could not remember everything that had been done to him. He knew he had been given barium through both ends, a CAT scan of the chest and abdomen, a bone marrow examination, and a liver biopsy. In addition, numerous tubes of blood had been drawn from his arm.

Meanwhile, to quiet his pain, he had been treated with a mild narcotic (hydromorphone), but the doses were ineffective, and although he complained constantly, his doctors refused to do anything about it. In fact, when Steve asked for a stronger narcotic, Dr. Prince told him he was not "going to make an addict out of him."

In addition to his reluctance to control the pain, Dr. Prince avoided reviewing the findings with Steve and Liz, although they begged him for detailed information. Days passed without a frank discussion. These were days during which Steve felt as if his life were ebbing. He had become listless and weak because he was unable to eat or sleep. He had no appetite. The aroma of food nauseated him. He had a constant burning pain that extended from his neck to his navel. No one seemed willing to give him relief.

"I was trained as an anthropologist," Steve said later. "Gathering information from key informants is an essential skill we learned in graduate school. I felt an urgency about my illness, as if my life depended upon gathering information as rapidly as possible. I used my skill to manipulate the doctors. I admit to being devious, but the straightforward approach had failed.

"So I'd say to the intern, 'The resident seems to think it's cancer.' Actually, the resident hadn't said anything, but it was a way of making the intern talk to me. Liz sat beside me with a note pad. She'd done graduate work in communication. We didn't miss a trick.

"After a few days, we had narrowed it down. The liver biopsy had been interpreted as adenocarcinoma. We forced Dr. Prince to commit himself. Finally, he deigned to give us an explanation, but he made it clear to both of us that the conversation was burdensome.

" 'It's quite serious,' Dr. Prince said. His long face telegraphed his feelings. 'There's no treatment. You have an extremely aggressive adenocarcinoma of the pancreas. I doubt you will live to see your baby.'

"When I asked him if I should be seen by an oncologist, he told me I had already been seen by one. Only then did I realize that the shy woman who had visited me earlier in the afternoon had been an oncologist. She had said nothing to me, just shook her head and left.

"Liz and I knew the situation was desperate. We had called around the city. By late the following afternoon we had obtained an oncology consultation from an expert at another university hospital. Adenocarcinoma is uncommon in young men, he told us. It rarely makes large masses in the chest. He asked my doctors to do another biopsy. Within twenty-four hours the diagnosis had been changed. I didn't have adenocarcinoma of the pancreas at all. I had lymphoma.

"I expected Dr. Prince to be delighted. There was a slim chance treatment might help me for a while. Instead, he seemed irritated by our interference in his 'management' of my case.

" 'You people are too involved for your own good,' he told us. 'You ought to leave your medical management to professionals.'

"I wanted to say, 'but we *have* relied on medical professionals. The oncologist from the other university is a department chairman. He also gave me *some* hope of survival. Pardon me for butting in on your work, sir, but *some* hope of living is better than what you were offering.' But I said nothing at all. I was in severe pain, deprived of sleep, weak, and anxious. But I had also endured hardships in the jungle of Brazil. And I had learned a lesson there: it would not improve my chance of survival to fight with Dr. Prince. Rather than make an enemy of him, I concealed my rage. Instead, I asked him if anyone was doing any research on lymphoma.

" 'Nope,' he said. 'You're not a whole lot better off with lymphoma than you were with adenocarcinoma. You're going to die anyway.'

"We were lucky. A network of friends had called around the city for us. Liz had collected several dozen references on lymphoma. Important work *was* being done only a few miles away. As unbelievable as it seemed, Dr. Prince had lied.

"Fortunately, the telephone was ringing off the hook by then. When the outside oncologist discovered the new diagnosis, he volunteered to help arrange a transfer to the research center where I could receive experimental treatments. The risk would be considerable, but I had a chance of cure.

"With certain death as the only other option, I was more than willing to take big risks. By then I could hardly sit up. I hadn't slept for two weeks. Dr. Prince, claiming he didn't want me addicted to narcotics, had reduced the doses of the hydromorphone. I had been in constant pain on full doses of the medicine, but with the lowered doses the pain had become excruciating.

"The rest you know. The treatment was intense, but I survived. After I stayed in remission for three years, they told me I was cured."

Steve and Liz are philosophical about Dr. Prince. They have forgiven him for making an incorrect diagnosis, for ordering tests without including them in the process, and for his reluctance to discuss the results with them. They have even forgiven him for being stingy with the pain medication.

"It may have been an honest difference of opinion," Steve said. "Although for the life of me I can't see why people with cancer should ever be left in pain because their doctors are worried about them becoming addicts."

It's harder to explain away Dr. Prince's excessive pride, his reluctance to seek opinions outside his institution when he had nothing useful to offer his patient.

"We live in an age burgeoning with medical information," Steve said. "All he needed to do was pick up the telephone, and he could have been a hero. He could have been honest when we asked if any research was being done on lymphoma. In spite of everything, we could have admired him if, instead of lying about it, he had just said, 'I don't know.' "

The uncertainty that applies to physical examinations and X-rays extends to all medical information. Scientific reports contain collected observations. The opportunity for error is manifold. Reviewers summarize scientific information in textbooks and journals. I have studied them in an attempt to better my understanding of oncology. The work is time-consuming and frustrating. Sometimes when I am finished reviewing a subject, I am less certain of the information than before I began to read about it. The data conflict with each other, the authorities disagree, the phenomena keep changing.

Among my colleagues, certainty is usually a sign of ignorance.

I was asked to deliver a lecture at a university cancer center. I had attended many lectures at the center, but I had never given one.

In the audience would be many academicians, people who would be more familiar with the subject than I was.

Months earlier, I had heard a talk on the same topic. It had been given by a world authority, a man who had performed studies in the area for more than thirty years. He had spoken with a dry sense of humor and a spellbinding style. Members of my audience who had heard his talk would be bored by mine, I feared.

In addition, experts had collaborated on two exhaustive reviews within the past year. I felt somewhat intimidated by the availability of individuals whose scholarly opinions carried far more weight than my simplistic views. The professional reviewers had taken a scholarly approach, whereas I could only read the material as a practitioner. I did not think a busy physician could prepare a lecture that could compete with such authorities for content or interest.

Although I continued to be fully occupied with my medical practice, I sought help from my hospital librarian and gathered a hundred recent articles on the topic. The deeper I got, the more aware I became of the complexity of the subject.

My preparation for the lecture was similar to my daily efforts to provide responsible information to my patients. As a practicing physician, I am confronted not with hundreds of articles but with tens of thousands. I cannot hope to know everything important in each of the pertinent articles about each disease I have to treat, yet I cannot take the chance of missing information that might help someone like Toby. If the literature contains information that will help save lives, reduce suffering, or improve human life, I want to know about it.

In the preparation of the lecture, I resisted the temptation to paraphrase the information in the review articles. If I were to deliver the lecture, I felt I should be ready to defend any statement I made. I forced myself to look at the primary data and to draw my own conclusions. I discovered I disagreed with the much-admired national expert. He had failed to answer a significant and obvious question in the course of his studies. In fact, he had failed to follow one of his own favorite principles: he had not used controlled trials to validate his findings. Without them his conclusions were suspect, no matter how great his authority.

To confirm my objections, I rechecked the details of dozens of reports. I could find no error in my thinking. To my chagrin, however, the professional reviewers had failed to emphasize the necessity of controlled trials. Although I did not know why they had been unwilling to criticize his work, I came to the conclusion that I would have to publicly disagree with him. With the papers in my hand, I raced into the kitchen where my wife was reading the newspaper.

"What do I do now?" I asked. "I don't dare disagree with a major authority. Should I ignore my own conclusions and just quote the information from the review articles?"

"I thought you had integrity," she said.

"But maybe I'm wrong," I said. "I have not yet read all the articles."

"You read the relevant ones, didn't you?"

"Several times."

"Then stick by your guns," she said.

A month later, as I approached the lectern at the cancer center, I wondered if it would be the last time I made such an appearance. Among the audience would be doctors who had spent their lives devoted to research projects of the sort I planned to discuss. I was afraid my criticisms would make me unwelcome.

As I turned to face the group, I saw among the audience interns, residents, and fellows. A thought came to me as I began to speak. Whatever the professors might think, I had an important message to give to those young physicians who were about to embark upon their careers in medicine. They had to know I was not afraid to challenge the authorities. I wanted young doctors to know that practicing physicians are willing to review a subject in depth, despite the effort and the scarcity of free time.

What followed, it turned out, was as revealing to the audience as it had been to me. My questions aroused interest in the academic community. Aware of the vitality of the intellectual exchange, I felt my efforts had proved worthwhile, not so much because of what I knew, but because of the questions I had been willing to ask. No one learned more from the lecture than I did.

I have become a teacher. When I was on a university faculty, I taught medical students and house officers. When I went into practice, I had to learn to teach people who knew much less about medical subjects, people who looked alarmed when I discussed sensitive topics. I could not assume they were familiar with the insides of the human body. We did not even speak the same language.

"Say it in English," Toby said with a chuckle.

"But I *did* say it in English," I thought to myself. I avoided medical terminology. I stuck to words whose definitions were common knowledge. I wondered where I had failed.

"The pleural space is the cavity between the lung and the chest wall," I said. "The lungs are like balloons. They expand and contract when we breathe. The sides of the lungs slide up and down within the chest cavity. The smooth surfaces of the pleural space make it possible to breathe without pain."

From Toby's questions I understood how difficult it was for him to comprehend what was so simple and obvious to me. The word *pleural* sounded strange on his ear. Before his illness he never heard it used. His knowledge of Latin was no help to him, for the word *pleura* comes from the Greek word "rib." Knowledge of the Greek word would not have helped him however, because the word *pleura,* as used in medicine, has nothing to do with ribs.

The pleural space is not a space, either. The two pleural surfaces—one on the outside of the lung, the other on the inside of the chest wall—are in direct contact, like an unopened plastic bag. It is possible to make a space by opening the chest, by putting air, or liquid, or solid masses between the two surfaces. But as it normally stands, there is no pleural space inside the chest.

As I told Toby these things, his eyes lit up. Without a firm grasp of the pleural space, he would not be able to understand where the liquid that had accumulated in his chest was located, why he was short of breath but not drowning. But my mind was miles ahead of his. I wanted him to know about the ways we could arrest the growth of his cancer, stop his symptoms. I felt as if I were giving a graduate lecture to a college freshman.

"I want to do everything I can to help myself," Toby told me. "I must understand my situation thoroughly."

I doubted he could reach his goal. It took years for me to accumulate my store of information. Even now the challenge boggles my mind.

Yet I was Toby's teacher. Like all committed teachers, I did not thwart my student's efforts to learn. Rather than force my knowledge on him, I waited for his questions. I wanted to enable him to feel he made his best effort. He was not a doctor and could never understand cancer the way I did, but he could have access to the information.

At dinner recently I sat opposite a man about my age. He was tall, lean, and redheaded. He looked serious but pleasant. I shook hands and introduced myself.

"What do you do?" he asked.

"I'm an oncologist," I said. "How about you?"

"I'm a prosecuting attorney," he said. "My name's Wright, and I usually am."

Silence followed.

"Showstoppers, aren't they?" he asked, suddenly laughing. "After we tell people what we do, conversation stops. No one wants to face me from the wrong side of the bench. Nobody wants to sit on the other side of your desk. I can only imagine how terrified I would feel if I had to see you as a patient."

"I try to keep the terror under control," I said. "The people who come to me want help. They didn't volunteer to have cancer, but many are determined to make the best of it. It's my responsibility to make it easier for them.

"I think we all feel better if we can laugh about something

before we start talking about cancer. It's easier to share something bitter after sharing something sweet. Children's drawings hang on the walls of my office, a reminder to me and my patients of the constant renewal of life."

I told the attorney about Brenda, a woman with lung cancer, who had been in my office recently. She knew her cancer was far advanced. At best she could stretch her life a few more months, but in those months another grandchild was due. She lived in expectation of welcoming a new member of the family, of seeing her daughter through her pregnancy. We had talked about her daughter's pregnancy with as much interest as we had talked about Brenda's cancer.

"But what do you tell people?" the attorney asked me. "I suppose they all say 'Tell me everything,' but you couldn't possibly tell them everything, even if you wanted to. Besides, I'm not certain I would want to know absolutely everything, just enough to make intelligent plans. How do you decide?"

It was his responsibility to prosecute criminals, but he was concerned about them. Although the suspects he had prosecuted were guilty of crimes, they had value as human beings, and he was concerned about the destructive effects of incarceration. Brutality of any kind offended him. Raw information about cancer, delivered without interpretation, seemed brutal to him because it could confuse, alarm, even destroy people.

"Do you think frightened people hear anything of what you have said?" he asked.

"They hear, but not everything. Fear confuses people. What they hear can be vastly different from what was meant. Repetition barely resolves the problem. Intelligence, preparation, patience, and reassurance do not guarantee clear understanding. Indeed, I've learned to expect most people to misunderstand at least part of what I say.

"I was not trained to talk to people about cancer. Rather, I watched many doctors doing it, each in a different way. Each patient was different, too, because each person has a different system of values, a different language, a different feeling about cancer. If I'm lucky, I'll learn something about the people before I talk to them. Otherwise, my task is much more difficult."

Three months after her mastectomy, a patient of mine named Mrs. Maynes consulted Dr. Felix about a minor problem. In the course of his examination, Dr. Felix performed a chest X-ray. Mrs. Maynes had an abnormality in her right lung.

"She could have metastatic cancer," he told his office nurse. "She needs a CAT scan of her chest. Get Mrs. Maynes on the telephone."

When the call was placed, Mrs. Maynes became alarmed.

"Why should I have a CAT scan?" she demanded of the nurse. In the background Mrs. Maynes could hear the nurse talking to Dr. Felix.

"The doctor says it will help us determine the cause of the abnormality on your chest X-ray. It could be something serious."

"What is that?" Mrs. Maynes asked.

"He can't say for certain, but he thinks it's important for you to have a CAT scan."

With some reluctance Mrs. Maynes allowed the nurse to schedule the CAT scan but not without letting her know she was furious with Dr. Felix. Aware of her distress, Dr. Felix called me.

"When I suggested a CAT scan, she became almost totally irrational," Dr. Felix told me. "See if you can settle her down. We don't want to ignore metastases. It may upset her to know, but it's better to do the scan now. I know you can't please everyone, but what are you going to do when people are irrational?"

I asked Mrs. Maynes to come to my office. "Bring all of your X-rays with you," I said. "I'd like to look at them before you have the CAT scan."

"I wasn't upset about the abnormal chest X-ray," Mrs. Maynes told me. "I was upset because he did not tell me himself. He made his nurse do it. I thought if there was something seriously wrong, he should have told me himself. I felt humiliated, as if I were a little child. Besides, he had not compared the new X-ray with my old ones. I wasn't certain he knew what he was doing."

Indeed, Dr. Felix had not reviewed Mrs. Maynes's previous X-rays. But only three months earlier, I had evaluated the abnormality on Mrs. Maynes chest X-ray in some detail. I had already done a CAT scan of her chest. I had concluded that there was nothing seriously wrong.

When Mrs. Maynes and I compared the new chest X-rays with those taken three months earlier, we could see no change in the dense area. We were both relieved.

Where did Dr. Felix go wrong?

The answer will be obvious to many nonphysicians and obscure to most physicians. Nonphysicians will wonder why Dr. Felix did not ask Mrs. Maynes if she were aware that her chest X-ray was abnormal. Doctors may wonder why he should have asked.

Yet Dr. Felix prevented himself from learning more about the problem when he asked his nurse to call Mrs. Maynes. He would have learned more if he had called her himself.

"Why didn't you tell the nurse you wanted to speak to Dr. Felix?" I asked Mrs. Maynes.

"Because I got excited," she told me. "No one realizes how scared I feel when people give me information about my cancer, especially over the telephone. Frightening information about my medical condition always befuddles me."

There is an ironic twist to the story. Dr. Felix's wife developed breast cancer later that year. She handled the information calmly, but he was terrified. His confusion clouded our discussion. I had to repeat myself many times before he could understand. After leaving the office, he would call at irregular hours with questions that had previously been answered.

I always showed him respect. Not because he was a doctor, but because he was in distress. That's when we need respect the most, and are least likely to receive it.

Help can come from unexpected sources. Great discoveries have come from relatively untutored people. People who did not know enough to understand that their ideas wouldn't work succeeded by sticking with them. In isolating insulin, for example, Banting and Best persisted in an experiment considered futile by seasoned academic physiologists. Purification of penicillin seemed an impossible chore to more "sophisticated" minds when Chain and Florey began the work. Clear thinking unclouded by prejudice is often required for new discoveries.

Margaret, a woman in her eighties, did not have much of a medical background. Although her mind was clear, deafness made her appear confused. She had a tendency to ramble. Yet despite her handicaps, she had a better idea of what was wrong with her body than the three physicians who had seen her before I did.

I remember the first time I heard about Margaret. Dr. Michaels, her family doctor, called me late one afternoon. There was a sense of urgency in his voice.

"My patient's bone scan showed metastatic cancer," Dr. Michaels said. "I found the report on my desk when I got back from vacation. I can't understand why nothing has been done. It's been three months."

"Where did the cancer start?" I asked.

"That's just it," he said. "We don't have a clue."

The three-month interval between the bone scan and his telephone call disturbed me. Before I saw Margaret, I wanted to understand the reason for the gap, if only to prepare myself for any anger she might feel at having her doctors delay so long in evaluating her for malignancy. For that reason, I called the other physicians who had seen Margaret while her doctor was away. The story gradually emerged.

Margaret had suffered from pain in her left hip. She had tried aspirin, but it was no help. She wanted to know whether something stronger might relieve her pain. She had taken a few medications, but when nothing helped, she went to an orthopedic surgeon. The orthopedist took X-rays of the hip and then a bone scan.

The radiologist knew nothing about Margaret when she looked at the bone scan. She saw abnormalities in three ribs and the left hip.

"In view of the widespread nature of the abnormalities, none of them in joints, a diagnosis of metastatic cancer seems most likely," the radiologist said in her report.

After hearing the report, the orthopedist told Margaret to return to Dr. Michaels. He mentioned that "something serious" was seen on the bone scan, but he did not tell her what it was.

Except for the pain in her left hip, which had finally begun to improve, Margaret felt well. Despite the scare the orthopedist had given her, she did not feel disposed to do anything about the abnormal bone scan. She had a lot of doctor bills already.

Margaret had lost twenty pounds and looked weary by the time she reached Dr. Michaels for an examination. Even after a thorough examination, the source of the cancer was not obvious. X-rays of her bowel and stomach, her breasts and chest, were all normal. No cancer was found on any of them.

"How can I help you?" I asked Margaret when she and her husband were seated in my office.

"First of all, I don't have cancer," Margaret said emphatically.

I nodded. It sounded like denial.

"What's wrong, then?" I asked.

"It's all because of my husband's prostate cancer," she said.

It seemed quite improbable to me, but I listened.

"The doctor found a cancer in his prostate, a small one. He told us they were common in people of his age. He's eighty-four. They gave him radiation treatments. That was no picnic."

"What does any of this have to do with Margaret's bones?" I wondered.

"After radiation therapy he had diarrhea. We live in an apartment. Before the radiation treatments he used to put the garbage in the incinerator. But he was afraid to go into the hall, so I had to do it myself.

"The door to the incinerator was difficult for me to manage with my hands full. One day I slipped, and the door slammed shut on me. I had several bruises.

"Because of the pain, it was hard to market or cook. My husband wouldn't eat, because food seemed to run right through him. We made do with soups and salads. I lost weight. Now the pain is better. I'm gaining some weight."

After listening to her story, I asked Margaret to identify the places where the door had struck her. The injured areas corresponded exactly to the places that had shown up on the bone scan. A current bone scan showed healing of the fractures and no signs of cancer.

Margaret's story was long-winded, but hers was the only one that mattered.

"He stood at the end of the bed and told me I had cancer," a patient wrote. "He told me dozens of little details I did not understand at all. He used words which sounded foreign. He told me not to worry. He said it was cancer, but that something could be done about it. But he never said whether I was going to die from it, which was all I wanted to know and the only thing that I could think about right then. He never asked me if I had any questions or took the time to listen to me tell him what was on my heart. Before I could say anything, he left the room. He seemed detached. It was as if he were announcing the results of an election or a football game. He did not seem to care about the content of his message."

I've let my patients teach me how to give them information. I've learned to ask if my timing is appropriate, whether they want signficant others to be there. Complaints cured me of talking about the good news and the bad news. I've been made to realize that my patients hang on every word and gesture; so I am careful of what I say and how I say it. I keep it simple.

I have learned to admit that I do not enjoy the business of delivering painful messages. I maintain eye contact. I mean what I say. I never lie.

No matter how clear the presentation, there is always a potential for misunderstanding. Instead of greeting misunderstanding with a sense of hopelessness, doctors and patients should accept the difficulty that comes with the exchange of information. Indeed, I think good communication is more technically difficult than delicate surgery. It takes more skill and patience, it is infinitely varied. No one ever finishes learning it. The need for it is endless. It cannot be scheduled or meticulously controlled.

Sterility improves the results of surgery. But communication between doctor and patient is killed by a sterile environment, free of the "contamination" of distraction and personality, rigidly cleansed of sentiment or humor, isolated from individual differences.

Evelyn had difficulty when I sent her to a consultant. She called me afterwards to complain about him.

"I picked the doctor for you because he is intelligent, compassionate, kind, and patient," I told her. "He enjoys a national reputation for expertise in his field."

From the silence on the telphone, I could tell that these characteristics had not won Evelyn's approval.

"He wouldn't tell me anything," she said. "He examined me. He had his technician run a lot of tests. He never discussed any of the results with me. He gave me an appointment to come back in a month and told me not to worry."

"What do you want to know, Evelyn?" I asked.

"I want to understand what's wrong with me," she said.

I could guess why the other doctor did not want to talk to Evelyn. She has difficulty formulating questions. She is quite forgetful and often repeats herself. She is eighty-two, and although she lives alone and drives a car, she is fearful that she may lose her independence because of her mental impairment.

I read the doctor's consultation note to her. She wanted me to explain each word in it, even the information I told her was not important because it had no impact on her health. She wanted to be in charge.

When I was done, she admitted her fear.

"I'm just an old lady who can't get anything straight," she said.

I knew better. Evelyn is not as quick as she once was, but she can understand if I am willing to take the time to explain everything in detail. She felt humiliated by the doctor who was impatient with her handicap. Before I hung up the telephone, I invited Evelyn to come to the office. I suspected she would have questions, some repetitious, about the information I had given her. The learning process takes time. I am prepared to spend it with her.

Peggy was fifty, a laboratory technician who understood a fair amount about medicine but had never been ill. A sudden episode of phlebitis prompted me to admit her to the hospital. Before she went home, I explained the use of coumadin, an anticoagulant that I expected her to take for the next six months.

"It's a complicated medication," I said. "It's quite safe if you follow the rules, but you must learn the rules before you go home."

I gave her detailed information, pausing after each statement for questions. I repeated the important points, using examples for clarity. I deliberately spoke in simple English. After the discussion I left the room, satisfied that I had done my job well.

The next day, when I visited Peggy in the hospital, her husband was at her bedside. I told him Peggy would be taking coumadin.

"What do we need to know?" he asked.

I waited for Peggy to repeat what I had told her the previous day. To my surprise, she could remember almost nothing of our discussion.

"I knew it yesterday," she said, laughing.

Even when presented in simple language, medical information is easy to forget. Apart from the factors that distract attention, learning about anatomy, physiology, pathology, and pharmacology strains the intellect. Medical students must constantly review. The best students forget more than they remember.

Physicians use words, phrases, and medical concepts in diverse ways. Fortunately, most illnesses require discussion with only one or two doctors. Cancer, however, is different. Patients with a single malignancy may have to contend with diagnostic and treatment information from many doctors, all strange to them. Discussions about a small breast cancer, for example, may involve discussions with a mammographer, a surgeon, a pathologist, a radiation therapist, a medical oncologist, a plastic surgeon, and the patient's primary physician. Each of the physicians has a separate but important message for the patient. Not infrequently, however, the messages appear to overlap and conflict. The resulting confusion adds to the anxiety. The anxiety is particularly aggravated by forcing people to make decisions based on confusing and conflicting information.

Vickie, who came to me for a routine physical, seemed to have a private vocabulary.

"Is there anything wrong?" I asked.

"I'm just getting old," she told me. "After all, I am eighty-two. When you're eighty years old, Doctor, there are bound to be things wrong. We just do the best we can."

"Yes, but was there some special reason why you came today?"

"I went to my old doctor once a year for a checkup. It had been a year since my last examination. I thought I should have a checkup."

"You have had no symptoms?"

"Nothing out of the ordinary."

After careful questioning I learned that she had some minor arthritic pain, occasional headaches, a mild degree of memory loss, and a weight loss of fifteen pounds.

"It's too much trouble to eat, Doctor. I need to have dental work. It's too hard for me to go the dentist."

"What about your bowel movements?" I asked.

"There's been some blood, she told me. "I have hemorrhoids."

There was more than blood. Vickie had a rock hard mass the size of a large apple in her rectum. I asked her if she was aware of it.

"Oh that," she said. "I had hoped you wouldn't examine me back there."

"But I always do. It's part of a complete physical examination."

"My other doctor never did that."

"Vickie," I said. "I have something troublesome to tell you. It may upset you to hear it, but it's better for you to know. I think you have a cancer."

"Maybe I'll die in my sleep," she said.

"Maybe not," I countered. "You might have a lot of pain if we don't take it out."

"I'm too old for surgery," she said.

"We've operated on people much older and sicker than you."

"Let me think about it," she said.

I saw her gaze shift as she spoke those last few words. After she left my office, would she tell anyone what I had said? Would she *really* think about doing something? Or would she go to bed each night hoping she would not wake up?

"Do you have children?" I asked.

"A son."

"Does he live near here?"

"Yes."

"Should I call him?"

"Don't do that. My granddaughter is having trouble with a pregnancy. My daughter-in-law is worried about her. I don't want to add to her burdens."

"They'll have to know sooner or later. Wouldn't it be better to inform them now?" I asked.

Vickie refused to let me call them. She gave a series of excuses. They were on vacation. They were busy with their own lives. She could handle this by herself. She had been a widow for thirty years. She was accustomed to her independence.

I understood my obligation to obey her wishes, but I was deeply disturbed about it.

Unless she died suddenly, if she did nothing about her cancer, she would probably suffer terrible pain and disability in the years ahead. I believed her pain and disability could be prevented or at least reduced. I did not know how to proceed.

Sitting around the Sabbath table, I asked my family what they would have done.

"It's her choice," one said.

"I'd call her son," said another.

"You have to persuade her," said a third.

Medical ethics are not theoretical concerns. They are at the root of hundreds of difficult decisions physicans make every day. Right answers do not exist. Yet we must find answers which seem right.

"One issue sways me," I said. "Despite saying she wanted to think it over, to wait awhile, to take care of her teeth first, she knew something serious was wrong. She did not refuse to let me do a rectal examination. She was not surprised when I found the cancer. Perhaps she had been unable to tell me what she wanted, but her body spoke for her. Some voice from deep inside of her cried out to me for help. I think I heard her inner voice, and I am going to answer it even if it means violating her expressed wishes. I think she's frightened and her fear has paralyzed her."

I called Vickie for a progress report each week. Each time I called, she had a new excuse for not taking action and not telling her son about the cancer.

"I don't know why I'm having so much trouble with it," she said. "Usually I am straightforward about problems. Don't worry, Doctor, I'll get to it."

Her description of herself as "different" convinced me to take the presumptuous step of informing her son about her cancer.

"I have violated her trust," I said. "I have never taken such liberties. I staunchly support privacy, but I believe my decision is in Vickie's best interest."

He listened thoughtfully while I explained the problem.

"What am I to do?" he asked when I had finished.

"Make yourself available. Ask about her health. Hint about your willingness to take her to doctors. Ask whether she has lost weight. Ask her if there is anything wrong."

"I'll try," he said.

A week later, I spoke with Vickie again. She mentioned nothing about a conversation with her son. I called him.

"She's clever, Doctor," he told me. "We asked her to come for dinner. We talked for two hours. We hinted heavily. She never acknowledged any problem."

I sighed. We had made our best efforts. They had failed. I continued to call every two or three weeks. She continued to delay.

Three months after her first visit, she came to my office.

"How are you doing, Vickie?" I asked.

"I'm here for a flu shot."

"But Vickie," I said, trying to sound sympathetic, trying to *feel* sympathetic, "having a flu shot and ignoring your rectal cancer is like swatting at flies when you have pigs in your living room. You're not going to save the carpet that way."

"I realize what you are saying, Doctor. I just can't do it."

"No, Vickie," I thought to myself. "You do not know what I am saying. We are talking different languages. When I talk of helping you, you do not understand. When I talk of ridding you of pain, of preventing disability, of treating you with dignity, of letting specialists find ways of relieving you of your distress, you do not understand me."

Months later, Vickie developed a high fever. In great distress, she called her son, who brought her to the emergency room. Until she arrived at the emergency room, nothing had been said about her rectal cancer. The emergency room doctor found her cancer had become infected. Vickie acted as if she knew nothing about the cancer.

Fluids and antibiotics helped to control the infection. A surgical specialist came to see her. With gentleness we listened.

"I know I was wrong not to do something about my cancer," Vickie kept repeating. "I don't know what came over me."

A biopsy showed she had cancer, but a CAT scan gave encouragement. The cancer had not spread beyond the pelvis. Curative treatment was still possible.

It is clear to many who practice medicine that a substantial number of people do not want to listen to medical information about themselves. Steve, the assertive young anthropologist who saved himself from dying of lymphoma, observed other patients on the cancer service.

"You could see the physicians were trying to tell the patients what was happening and the patients were tuning them out. Their eyes would roll back, and their expression would turn flat. They did not want to know."

In this regard, I have a confession to make. Only with great difficulty can I listen to medical information about myself. Despite my eagerness to communicate medical information to others, I prefer not to look at my own chest X-rays and laboratory data. During several minor illnesses I have let my doctors bear the weight of the responsibility for making decisions. I accept their judgments even when they disagree with mine. I have chosen my physicians carefully. They are meticulous, thoughtful, sensible, and informed. They have a sense of humor. I have wanted them to bear the weight of caring for me without making me aware of the burden.

My confession is intended to reassure others who share with me the desire to allow our physicians to make our medical decisions. Neither ignorance nor medical incompetence has led us to delegate this awesome responsibility to a trusted physician. We are aware of the potential for bias if we attempt to be objective about ourselves. When our lives are at stake, we prefer to delegate management to a "detached" expert.

Our physicians should give us detailed explanations, even if they are painful. Our reluctance to listen should not excuse our physicians from seeking to inform us. So remember these lines, Bob (my physician), if and when you have momentous news for me. Then the grins we exchanged across your desk as we joked about the vagaries of the health care system will have to give way to the painful and distressing news about my body. And though I rage and cry, I will want to know what you think is wrong and what you want to do about it.

When people come to me with notebooks full of references, with legal pads and tape recorders, with lists of questions and with witnesses who are expected to judge my performance, I am grateful for the opportunity to teach them about their illnesses, to share information, and to test the accuracy of their knowledge before they leave my office.

When people come with blank faces, no questions, and a seeming indifference to the messages I believe they should acquire, I try doubly hard to gain their attention. I take notes and give them copies to take home. I draw pictures. I tell stories. I do not always succeed, but I am always willing to try.

I know there must be reasons why people digress, but I do not always learn what they are. I am particularly mindful of Jerry, a practicing attorney, who had myeloma. When he saw me, he rarely talked about his malignancy. Instead, he told me about malpractice cases he was pursuing against physicians. I wondered silently if he was trying to transfer his anxiety to me. If so, he sometimes succeeded. Some of his clients were suing physicians for whom I had great respect. I did not think I should be privy to the information he insisted on relaying in great detail. Yet this same attorney, when confronted with equally detailed information about myeloma, turned it away.

"I can't handle it," he said.

I suspected he was correct. He feared he would lose his law practice, even his girlfriend, if anyone knew he had myeloma. He wanted to keep his myeloma a secret from them. But he wanted to keep it a secret from himself as well.

"I've seen a number of professional people who continued to

work despite their cancers," I said. "In fact, our president had cancer. It didn't detract from his activities."

"But his cancer was cured, Doctor. You told me mine could not be cured."

"There are many diseases that can't be cured, Jerry," I said. "People learn to live with them."

It took two months for Jerry and me to learn to talk about his myeloma using terms with which we both felt comfortable. I learned it was *his* role, not mine, to remind himself that he was sixty-five and his best years were behind him. *He* could say he felt well, continued to be full of life, and might live another decade with his myeloma. It was *my* role to tell him the laboratory values, to remind him of hopeful information. It was *his* role to tell me he believed meaningful relationships meant more than power and money. *He* could tell *me* he had learned to love a woman in other ways than having sex with her. It was *my* role to listen to his philosophy, admire his obvious talent as an attorney, even to hear him brag about his prowess as a plaintiff's attorney in medical malpractice cases.

There are ironies that doctors have to face in "communicating" with their patients. Giving careful attention to a problem sometimes produces more confusion than clarity. Justin, a patient of mine with lymphoma, could barely talk to me about his cancer, although both of us engaged in a serious effort. Luck and mutual desire helped us succeed.

He had lymphoma in his upper arm, an unlikely place for such a swelling. Indeed, its unusual appearance had caused his doctors to attribute it to an injury and to ignore it while they searched elsewhere for the cause of his lack of appetite and abdominal pain. By the time I first saw him, a variety of physicians had devoted expensive attention to every other part of his body even though he initially complained of a painful lump in his right arm. Not until he was seen by a department chairman at a university did anyone suggest a biopsy of the painful lump. But that simple twenty-minute procedure ended a six-week ordeal of diagnostic uncertainty. Justin's distrust of the medical establishment had honest origins.

Our early attempts at communication succeeded with deceptive ease. He brought with him the documents from the university. The written information freed me from the burden of prying loose the facts about the evolution of his illness. In some detail he told me about his angry encounters with several of his physicians. He even offered gratuitous suggestions about orifices into which they might insert their instruments. But about his clinical course he provided little insight, and as a consequence, I did not at first know how reticent he was about his medical problems.

Justin took chemotherapy for several months. The lump in his arm disappeared quickly, then quickly returned. He was given radiation therapy. The lump in his arm vanished again, but he developed lumps in his neck. A new form of chemotherapy was started. His lumps disappeared again.

One day he called me in moderate distress. He had a pain in his right side. It wasn't severe, but it was constant. Pain medication had not helped. In addition, he had diarrhea. I queried him about fever, change in diet or urination, a history of surgery for appendicitis. He denied any of these. I was tempted to treat him by telephone, but a sixth sense made me ask him to come to the office. In no way did he communicate alarm, a sense of severity, or a fear his pain might augur some dire complication of his illness.

Before I examined him, I ordered laboratory tests. He balked at my aggressiveness, claiming I did too many blood tests. I countered that the laboratory tests were essential for making diagnoses. I needed my tools to help me decide what to do.

While the blood word was being done, I asked him dozens of questions. His answers to them were generally negative. Suddenly, from deep inside my brain, a recollection came floating back. I remembered that his left kidney had been removed some forty years earlier. In a flash the diagnosis became obvious. His right kidney was blocked with a stone. The pain he might have been expected to feel had been blunted because of kidney failure.

"Why didn't you remind me you only had one kidney?" I asked, explaining that, except for my sudden recollection, I might have missed the diagnosis.

"Why should I?" he asked. "I told you that last year." Then came the killer: "You're my doctor."

I was grateful for the sense of trust Justin had in me, but no human being can remember every bit of information about each patient. I need prompting.

The road to insanity is paved with musings about close calls and possible failures. Even so, the mystery of my communication with Justin deepened. He later told me he had suspected his right kidney was blocked when the pain first started, *but he never said so.*

"I wanted to find out what you thought," he said. "I wanted you to have an open mind. I was afraid my opinion might have an undue influence on you."

Information flows at different rates in different environments. We cannot speed its transmission by willpower alone. Cooperation and a bit of luck are needed.

Recently, I was asked to care for Edith, an eighty-four-year-old woman, when my partner left on vacation. In addition to having lung cancer, she was depressed, arthritic, and the survivor of two heart attacks. In addition to these daunting problems that frustrated management of her cancer, she had poor vision and was deaf. When I arrived, her chief concern was nausea and vomiting.

In the brief space of a fifteen-minute hospital visit, it was my responsibility to communicate to Edith that her doctor was away for two weeks, a surgeon would be discussing the risks of operating on her lung cancer, and I would be caring for her symptoms. In fact, the principal purpose of my visit was to diagnose the cause of her nausea and vomiting.

Because of her deafness, I sat beside her, near the window, and slowly enunciated each word. It took time to deliver my messages and to listen to her responses. She told me other doctors (not my partner) had given up communicating with her and spoke with her sister instead. Edith had become incensed at being omitted from direct exchange with her doctors, even though her sister was supportive and interested.

After I was finished with the slow delivery of information, I paused for questions. Edith spoke as if she had understood almost nothing of what I had said. Instead, she commented on the nurse's clothes as if she were avoiding me.

"You didn't even thank me for taking extra time with you," I said.

"You weren't any help," she said. "I can't see your mouth because you are in front of the window and the light is too bright. I can't hear you, either. Your voice is too harsh because you talk too loudly. I can understand better if you speak more softly."

I knew I would be late for the office if I stayed, but I did not want to leave the room without giving Edith a chance to understand me. I moved to the other side, spoke softer, and let her ask questions. Before I left, she thanked me twice.

Science has revolutionized medicine but simple courtesy can unravel some problems more successfully than molecular biology.

9
BATTLES

BUILT into our culture is a love of victory. Never mind the glorious hero who sacrificed everything for a cause, forget the courageous politician who risked his career for a principle, ignore the athlete who excelled in every way but one: his score was second best. At bottom, many of us only want to know who won.

In July of 1980, Bjorn Borg defended his Wimbledon title against John McEnroe. It was one of the most magnificent tennis matches I have ever watched, a full five sets, the final set taking many extra games. More was at risk than the gold cup. Borg was reaching for a record: five consecutive Wimbledon titles. Clearly older, less energetic than McEnroe, his strategy would hinge on the essential qualities of a great athlete: self-control and concentration. Borg was a consummate master of both. Since his early teens McEnroe had set his sites on beating Borg. Despite his temperament, McEnroe had superb mastery of the game and power to match. Their battle held me spellbound for hours until, at last, Borg won. As is the custom, McEnroe was approached for comment. I longed for him to say, "That was fantastic! No matter how many titles I win in the future, I will never play a more exciting match." Instead he said, "I lost," as if winning were the only thing that mattered.

Time has been kind to John McEnroe. Not only did he go on to win Wimbledon three times, but at the age of thirty-three he reached the semifinals, losing only to the tournament champion, André Agassi, whose grass-game victory owed much to McEnroe's coaching. More gracious in defeat in 1992 than he was in 1980, McEnroe talked about the good feeling of playing great tennis rather than the sting of losing an important match.

McEnroe is an exception to a trend in modern competition. Too many contemporary athletes continue to ignore Grantland Rice's couplet,

> When the One Great Scorer comes to write against your name,
> He marks—not that you won or lost—but how you played the game.

As spectators, we have difficulty appreciating the culmination of years of practice, the care, the effort of athletes competing in world-class events. We are too like the commentators, ignoring their magnificent performances as we concentrate upon their scores.

"Who got the gold?" we ask, oblivious to the fact that only fractions of a second separated the victor from an impressive cohort of competitors. In a sense, they *all* got the gold, and we missed it.

Unfortunately for us, our attitude about competitive sports often translates into rules of life. We strive to dominate rather than negotiate. We retain control instead of sharing it. We "plan" our lives instead of developing relationships. We strive to win the battle against cancer instead of accepting the limitations of our bodies.

I am not a nihilist. I believe in making a maximal effort to cure cancer. I use every device at my disposal to eliminate cancer cells in order to restore my patients to their previous states of health. I feel a sense of triumph when treatment succeeds.

But just as I do not try to make the blind force themselves to see or the deaf strain to hear or people with Alzheimer's disease make a "sincere effort to remember," I don't insist that people with cancer fight a battle I know they cannot win. People who insist they or others should "fight cancer" ought to pause a moment to consider who or what the enemy is.

Rex Kane was a superb athlete, sportsmanlike, competitive, and able to concentrate all his energy on winning. He was also a young man with a disease that should have been curable.

When Rex was a college freshman, he had no thought of dying. In fact, he had never been ill. Like many young people, Rex thought cancer was a disease other people got. Consequently, he ignored his symptoms: a dwindling appetite and loss of weight.

"Too much exercise and rotten dormitory food," he told his father. "That's why I'm getting thinner. If you were eating it, you'd lose weight, too."

"But you've been home three days, and you've eaten less than I have," his father said.

"I probably have a bug of some sort, Dad. I've had a fever. At night I wake up drenched with sweat. I'll get better."

"Why don't you drink beer any more?"

"I can't, Dad. Something strange happened months ago. When I tried to drink beer, my back hurt. My potassium must be low."

"Your potassium? Does that cause pain?"

"One of the guys in the dormitory said it does."

Rex and his father remembered the conversation a month later. They were in his doctor's office one Friday afternoon. Rex had noticed something new, a lump on the left side of his neck.

"Weight loss, sweats, a lump in your neck and alcohol intolerance," his doctor said. "It sounds like Hodgkin's disease."

With practiced fingertips the doctor explored the recesses of Rex's body, looking for enlarged lymph nodes. He found nodules the size of walnuts on both sides of Rex's neck.

"He'll need a biopsy," the doctor said.

The hospital required Rex to have a chest X-ray before the biopsy. He had a cauliflower-sized shadow in the center of his chest. The doctor was startled by the size of the shadow because Rex had no cough or shortness of breath.

A surgeon biopsied a lymph node from Rex's neck.

"It's Hodgkin's disease," the pathology department reported. "Mixed cellularity."

Sitting at a microscope with Rex's internist, the surgeon examined the lymph node. There was no doubt about the diagnosis. "How far has it spread?" the internist asked.

"It's in his neck and chest, John. We did a CAT scan of his abdomen. His spleen is enlarged. He has lymph nodes along his aorta."

"That's stage III," the internist said.

"At least stage III-B," the surgeon said. "He has had fever, chills, sweats, and weight loss. It may even be stage IV-B when we have more information."

"What are his chances?"

"He wants to know the same thing," the surgeon said. "I've been told he has an 80 percent chance of permanent remission."

"That's encouraging. I can guess what his parents are feeling." The internist sighed.

In silence, the surgeon heard the sigh. He suspected the internist was thinking about his own dead son. The two of them had often sailed together on Chesapeake Bay. The boy had been bright and handsome, tragically snatched from life in his late teens. In the years that followed, when the surgeon and the internist talked about a serious illness in a young person, the boy's spirit seemed to hover over them.

"When our children die, we never finish grieving," the surgeon thought. He put his hand on the internist's shoulder.

"We're going to do our best," he said.

The internist smiled sadly.

Rex took the news remarkably well. He understood he had a form of cancer. He recognized the possibility of death.

"It's dangerous but curable. What do I do about it?" he asked.

"We can't cut it out," his oncologist told him. "It's too far spread for radiation. We're going to use chemotherapy. Six months ought to do it."

His father smiled in the background. Rex looked serious but calm.

"I'm not weak, Doctor," he said. "Even with the fever, weight loss, and fatigue, I can still play eighteen holes of golf. I cried last night, but I am never going to cry again. I'm going to lick this thing."

When he first came to our office, Rex was regularly seen by one of my colleagues. Even though I was not caring for him at the time, I could not help noticing him because he was much younger than most of our other patients. He looked strangely out of place with his youthful skin and powerful build. His golden hair, which he never lost, had an almost regal sheen. He surveyed the territory with cerulean eyes set in a handsome face.

Rex took his chemotherapy while perched in a position from which he could view the entire office. As I went about my work, I felt his probing eyes staring at me, as if he could enter my mind and analyze my thoughts. I felt my professional detachment weaken under the power of his gaze.

While chemicals dripped into Rex's veins, he played chess with his father. The two of them acted as if they were waiting out a storm at the airport. The chemotherapy seemed irrelevant to their relationship.

"Put your knight on queen's bishop six, and you're a dead man in three moves," I heard Rex say when they were midway through a game.

"Damn, you beat me again!" his father exclaimed. "Who the hell taught you to play?"

"It's like math, Dad," Rex replied. "You have to think."

"I'm no slouch at chess," Henry Kane told me. "But Rex makes me look like a beginner. Even with all the medication, he can still beat me."

As the months passed, Rex was often seen in our office. We reacted to his presence as if he were part of our family. When he bounced into the laboratory in pursuit of his tests, we reveled in his resilience. His blood counts were never low.

The intense gaze that pierced my emotional armor became a part of my life. His yearning to survive warmed my heart when he visited our office. When our eyes met, I felt as if we spoke wordless paragraphs in an instant, as if we were linked like arm wrestlers, intent on testing each other's strength.

Weeks passed. My colleague ordered CAT scans of his chest and abdomen. The Hodgkin's disease had disappeared.

"It looks like you're in remission," my colleague said. "How do you feel?"

"I'll feel better when I break eighty," Rex replied. "I shot eighty-two last week."

The remission lasted only six months. The oncology nurse was the first to notice the signs of relapse.

"I don't like the look of his face," she said to me one day. "There's something wrong. I can't tell you what it is. Rex is not well. His doctor will be gone for several weeks. He asked that you take care of Rex until he returns."

"I feel fine," Rex told me.

"Then why do you complain of pain in your left side?" I asked.

"It's indigestion," Rex said.

The nurse was unconvinced.

A month later, Rex returned. This time the evidence was plain. The night sweats had returned. His appetite was gone. He had lost eight pounds.

Although I could not find any signs of Hodgkin's disease with my fingers, I was worried. We ordered additional CAT scans. When I reviewed them with the radiologist, I was shocked.

My mouth felt dry as I prepared to talk with Rex and Henry in my office.

"What did the CAT scan show?" he asked.

"It isn't good," I said.

"You mean, it's relapsed," he said.

I was surprised to hear him use the technical word. I nodded.

"What do we do now?" Rex asked.

"We should start more chemotherapy."

"I want to live, Doctor. Whatever it takes, let's do it."

I helped the Kanes obtain second opinions at several cancer centers. Before we started the second course of chemotherapy, Rex had seen or spoken with four experts in the field. All the other oncologists agreed with my advice. I arranged for Rex to receive more chemotherapy.

Again I felt the haunting power of his eyes while the chemotherapy coursed his veins. He seemed to have concentrated his physical strength within his head, as if his mind could destroy his Hodgkin's disease. Like David with his slingshot, he stood his ground against a mighty force.

Rex changed. He acted more worldly than his college classmates. His step lost its bounce. His lightheartedness gave way to somber thoughtfulness. He had the manner of a person twice his age.

He wrote an article for the school newspaper in which he described his struggle. He compared himself to a prizefighter who continued to battle even when he knew he could not win. The crowd cheered as he struggled with his opponent. Valiantly he resisted defeat. He gloried in the crowd's enthusiasm. Rex knew he was unlike a boxer, however. Even after defeat, a boxer could plan a comeback. If Rex lost this fight, there would be no others.

As if his mind commanded his body, all the signs of Hodgkin's disease disappeared. No longer able to smile with simple optimism about his chance for cure, Rex greeted me with studied concern when he returned to my office for examinations.

"What do you think?" I asked him.

"I shot eighty-one last Saturday," he said. "And I wasn't half trying."

In three weeks he was back.

"You're early," I said.

"I found another node," he said.

I confirmed his report.

"This is starting to look serious," he said, but his eyes were twinkling.

His father, tense but faithful, sat poised with notebook in hand.

"We'll need more opinions, I suppose," he told me.

Once again, we called cancer centers around the country. Evidence showed some hope for transplantation with Rex's own bone marrow.

"You could give him higher doses of chemotherapy," an investigator told me. "It's his only hope. Of course, it won't work if he has Hodgkin's disease in his bone marrow."

"He didn't in the past."

"Do another two samples," he told me. "Just to be sure."

Rex, Mr. Kane, and I sat in my office late one May afternoon, Mr. Kane had his notebook open. As we spoke, he checked off questions, wrote down answers. In the course of learning about his son's illness, Mr. Kane had developed a remarkable facility with medical language. Rex seemed detached, as if he were a physician rather than a patient.

"You've gone from 80 percent chance of cure to less than twenty."

"Whatever chance is left, it's all I've got."

"The price of cure may be quite high," I said.

"I don't care if it's a million dollars," Rex said. "It's my only life. It's worth it to me."

"I was thinking of the physical and emotional cost," I said.

I took specimens of bone marrow from both sides of his pelvis. I could feel him tense as I used pressure to pierce his tough bones, but he did not complain. He was breathing rapidly, but I assumed he was anxious.

"We'll need to talk some more," I said. "Come back in two days. I want to have an opportunity to examine your bone marrow under the microscope."

To my surprise, Rex was back the following day.

"I can't breathe," he said.

He was pale, weak, and breathing rapidly. His temperature was 103°. A chest X-ray showed fluffy infiltrates in both lungs. I admitted him to the hospital.

The next day, I received a call from Dr. Johns, a consulting lung specialist. He delivered a terse message.

"If you don't do something about Rex this afternoon, I think he will be dead in the morning."

"What about the lung biopsy?" I asked. "What kind of infection does he have?"

"It's not an infection, Dan," he said. "It's Hodgkin's disease."

I felt as if I had been kicked in the stomach. Rarely have I seen Hodgkin's disease spread into the lungs like pneumonia. For Rex to suffer from another rare event seemed horribly unfair.

"How stupid of me," I thought. "I know life isn't fair."

I dashed to the hospital where I found Rex, propped up in bed, ghostly white and gasping for breath. Oxygen, administered by nasal prongs, did not relieve him. His family had gathered around his bedside. His father sat in a corner with his head down. His brother, David, knelt beside him, holding his hand. Mrs. Kane greeted me when I arrived.

"Is there anything you can do?" she asked.

I did not want Rex to die of Hodgkin's disease. His disease had progressed despite everything we had done. No degree of effort had been spared by Rex, his family, or the medical community. He had received maximal doses of medication. He had fought with courage and determination. And yet, unless I could pull some miracle out of an almost empty hat, Rex would be dead by the following afternoon. I was scared.

I reviewed the clinical data. The chest X-ray was clouded with progressive Hodgkin's disease. A band of white fuzz spread across his lung fields. Only his physical strength enabled him to continue breathing. I knew his endurance would not last. Worn out by the effort of breathing, he would die of exhaustion.

Rex had been treated with ten different chemotherapeutic drugs by then. His Hodgkin's disease had become resistant. Radiation therapy was out of the question. We did not have time to seek out experimental therapies. Mrs. Kane searched my face, her pleading eyes asking if I were aware of some helpful plan of treatment. Unfortunately, I wasn't.

I surveyed the Kanes. Rex looked numb, almost unaware of his surroundings.

"You are gravely ill," I said. "I must take drastic action."

"What are you going to do?" Rex asked.

No standard therapy had been developed for such a predicament. I racked my brain for alternative methods I might use. Very little came to mind. I felt as if Rex and I were speeding down white-water rapids in a canoe without paddles.

I never dared hope that he would live much longer after that. Death from Hodgkin's disease was a virtual certainty for Rex. But I found myself swept up in Rex's unquenchable thirst for life. I did not want to watch him die. I wanted to see him laughing in my office, not languishing in bed. I wanted him to breathe freely, not gasp for air like a marathon runner in the final miles of a race. I did not want to be forced to live with the memory that Rex had died while he was in my care, that I had forced him to accept what for him was unacceptable. His eyes had done their work on me. I felt as if part of him were within me, directing my decisions, compelling me to succeed.

Rex's brother David knelt at his bedside. Like a supplicant, he clutched Rex's hand. Until that afternoon, I had never met David. Of all those in the room, he seemed to be most tightly bound to Rex, still holding on when the rest of the family appeared to recognize approaching death. His face revealed a mixture of pleading and distrust, or rather a willingness to trust so long as the outcome was favorable.

"I hope you know what you're doing," David said.

My stomach tightened as he ignited my own anxieties. Would David be willing to concede that I "knew what I was doing," if nothing I did was helpful? I looked toward Rex's father. Seated in the corner, he refused to make eye contact with me. His notebook lay on the floor, unopened.

"Give me some comfort, Henry," I wanted to say to him. "I, too, have a son. If you were the doctor and my son were dying, I'd forgive you for not being able to save him."

He seemed to be too overcome with pain even to acknowledge my presence.

I nodded to Mrs. Kane as I prepared to leave the room. Wordlessly, she followed me into the hallway. As she came, I saw Rex's fifteen-year-old brother, Michael, emerge from the shadows. Michael was taller than Rex and resembled his mother. Despite his callow slenderness, I saw echoes of Rex's features in his nose and chin. In place of Rex's serious expression, an earnest sweetness suffused Michael's placid face.

Henry had appeared to be the strongest member of the family. Calm and methodical, he analyzed every problem. He kept notes, organized his thoughts, asked intelligent questions. At this, the toughest moment we had faced thus far, he remained silent. It was Mrs. Kane who emerged from the shadows prepared to cope with the situation.

As we stood in the hall, weighing the imponderable, I began to feel this mother's strength and the calm steadiness of her youngest son. Like faithful pilgrims supported by unshakable faith, they steadied each other. Michael's presence reminded his mother of her obligation to be a model for him; her gentle strength quieted his fears.

"Before you speak," she said dry-eyed, "please understand that I know that you cannot control what happens."

"Thank you," I said, realizing I was on the verge of tears. "I would rather someone else were here in my place."

"Life has a way of playing tricks on us."

"I have no way of knowing what to do for him."

"I'm not surprised. He's very ill."

"It might be possible to shrink the Hodgkin's disease. Of course, it would only be temporary."

"His father needs more time," Mrs. Kane said quietly. "I know what's coming. Do what you can."

Not certain what I could accomplish with more chemotherapy, I started to turn away. My sagging shoulders must have revealed my feelings.

"One more thing," I heard her say. I turned to face her.

"What's that?" I asked.

"I think you need one of these." She stretched up on her toes and locked me in a tight embrace.

I decided to give Rex cyclophosphamide. I gave him a substantial dose. Twice in the past I had used it in similarly severe situations. I understood the risk. It might help him, but it probably would not. I could think of nothing else that would give him a reasonable chance of surviving until the morning. I relayed instructions to the pharmacy. Armed with a syringe filled with the drug, I reentered Rex's room. I sat at his bedside and slowly injected the medication into Rex's intravenous line. I saw David stir.

"By the way," he asked, "what did the bone marrow show?"

I looked at him, wishing he had not asked. It was too late. Rex opened his eyes just wide enough to allow our eyes to meet.

"It had Hodgkin's disease in it," I said. Rex's strength seemed to ebb under the force of those words.

"Then it's hopeless!" David gasped.

"Let's see what this will do," I pleaded. It seemed like the wrong time to talk about Rex's future prospects.

I could not sleep that night.

The next morning, I postponed visiting Rex until I had seen my other patients. When I reached his room, I was amazed. The oxygen was off. He was sitting on the side of his bed playing chess with David.

"I've got two strokes to go!" he said.

Two weeks later, Rex shot seventy-nine.

A month passed before we could speak to each other about the dramatic episode in the hospital.

"You saved my life," Rex said. We were sneaking cookies from the office pantry.

"I know," I said, feeling a tremendous weight. I remembered a Chinese proverb that warned that if you save a person's life, he or she becomes your permanent responsibility. I felt the weight of Rex's life as if it were mine to preserve. "I am not certain I could do it again."

"I don't like that kind of talk," Rex said.

"Neither do I," I said.

I began this chapter with a declaration that death is not defeat, nor life a victory. We live by virtue of conditions largely beyond our control. When malignancy, like Hodgkin's disease, fails to yield to our interventions, no power of mind, no effort of will enables us to prevail.

People close to Rex heard a strident cry from a youth who had much in him. The reverberation of the cry lasted long after the voice was stilled. Rex had a wealth of creative energy, a powerful imagination, a keen intelligence, and a relentless objectivity about himself. Those characteristics screamed for expression before their owner perished.

A few years have passed since Rex died. I am older if not wiser. I have counseled many when death became inevitable. I've learned to talk of peaceful death as if I understood what it meant. And slowly, because it hurts to think about it, I have learned that some people do not achieve a peaceful death. Their yearning, their energy, their tenacious hold on life persists despite advancing cancer. Too open-eyed to ignore the reality of fatal illness yet too stubborn to accept its finality, they strive to live, screaming at nature turned awry, even until their last breaths.

Thus it was with Rex, who sought to separate his vibrant, vital self from the Hodgkin's disease that had sneaked inside of his body and destroyed it from within. In the fifteenth round of a world-class championship fight, Rex went down swinging, still trying to rise from the mat before the referee reached ten. If willpower alone decided survival, Rex could have lived to be a hundred and twenty.

Much as I tried to lead Toby in the direction of acceptance, for him life was victory, and death defeat. Like a contemporary athlete, he could not accept defeat, even though his cancer had progressed. Lacking an effective treatment, we continued to battle together long after "victory" had become impossible.

"I can't breathe!" Toby told me during an urgent telephone call one afternoon.

"You mean you're short of breath," I said. "How long has it been a problem?"

"About three hours," he said. I could hear the pitch of his voice rise as he spoke, the words coming in short phrases interrupted by whistling sounds.

"We'll move you to the hospital."

Within the hour, I met him in the emergency room. At first glance, his appearance had not changed since our previous meeting two weeks earlier. He still had tanned skin, a gleaming eye, and an easy laugh. A casual observer might have sent him home. While we talked, I counted his respirations.

"I always feel better when I see you," he said.

"I feel the same way when I see my doctor," I told him.

At rest, without talking, his respirations were about twenty-four a minute, not fast enough to indicate serious difficulties, but faster than normal. His pulse had increased, too. His lungs were compromised.

"Do you think it could be fluid?" Toby asked. "It was fluid the last time."

"Maybe," I said.

I ordered a chest X-ray and examined it closely with the radiologist.

"It could be anything," the radiologist said, sucking on his red china marker. "The left side of his chest is almost completely opaque, but it has not changed in six months. The right side has scattered densities. They could be fluid, scars, or metastatic cancer." He indicated suspicious areas with the marker. "Those look more like cancer, but the others look more like fluid. Sorry. I guess I'm not much help to you."

"On the contrary," I told him, "As long as there's a possibility of helping him by removing extra fluid, we'll try it." Toby glowed when I gave him the news. As always, a ray of hope could illuminate his world for days. After treatment with a potent diuretic, his breathing improved. By the end of the week, he could walk to the bathroom without assistance and even venture short distances into the hall. He felt comfortable without the oxygen streaming into his nostrils. Each day he seemed a little stronger, a little more optimistic.

When the weekend arrived, his family converged from Florida, Ohio, and New York. For the first time, I met his son, Toby Thompson, Jr. Like his father, he was slim and animated. His calm demeanor and self-confidence conveyed an image of the sort of strength that does not need to advertise itself. He was responsible for a major project from which he could be spared but briefly. I learned little else about him.

Julie, the daughter who worked with the hospice society, wanted to come to terms with her father's illness.

"Don't you think it's time to make a statement about my father's prognosis, Doctor?" she asked. "Mother needs help in the home. She doesn't complain, but she has macular degeneration. She has difficulty reading, especially at night. If we ask the hospice society to help, it will reduce the strain on her."

She paused and looked at me expectantly.

"Someone will have to tell him he's dying," she said.

Silence surrounded me.

I postponed discussion while I used a potent diuretic to force the fluid out of his lungs. Each day I hoped his weight would drop as evidence that the diuretic might have worked. When his weight ceased to fall, I knew further efforts with diuretics would not help. I repeated the chest X-ray. It had not changed. Two options remained: tell Toby that medications would not help his lungs, or hide behind a lie. I was ready to ask the hospice society for help.

"Do you want me to tell him that his time is short?" I asked Ginny.

"Not if it means destroying his hope," she said firmly.

I winced. To obtain hospice care meant telling Toby he had a life expectancy of less than six months. But Ginny believed Toby could not accept the prospect of so short a life span. He continued to talk about living for years and to make plans for "when he got well." Whenever I asked him if he wanted more facts, he refused.

To preserve his spirit, I would have to tell him about his life expectancy without destroying his dreams. I asked Ginny to meet me in Toby's room the following morning to provide moral support.

"I'd like to send you home, Toby," I said.

"Do you think I'm ready?" he asked. Once again, his face looked tense. "I don't want to make another trip to the hospital in an ambulance. Will I need oxygen? How can I manage if I need a shot in a hurry? In the hospital I can push a call button. In minutes I am surrounded by nurses who always seem to know exactly what to do for me. Ginny doesn't know much about nursing."

"But, Toby," I said, "I can arrange to have it all at home. A special bed. Oxygen. Shots. Even a call button."

"Really, Doctor? Will it be as good as the hospital? Will everything work? Will it cost a fortune? I'm not made out of money, you know."

"Your insurance will cover most of it, Toby. The people who will come are trained professionals. They use hospital equipment."

"There's got to be a catch."

For a moment I could not speak. Thoughts flew through my mind. I struggled to maintain eye contact with Toby as I wrestled with myself.

"You will have to sign a paper, Toby," I said. My voice cracked.

"What? Why?"

"The people who will come belong to hospice."

"I thought I was going home. I'd rather stay in the hospital. Isn't a hospice like a nursing home, but worse?"

"Your home will be your hospice. It's the best place for you now."

"Why do you need my signature?"

"It's a technical matter. We don't know any more about the future now than we did yesterday, Toby. But your insurance will pay for the hospice only if I tell them your life expectancy is six months or less. Don't ask me why. It's the same for everyone."

My words were flowing a bit too fast. I wanted to get past this point painlessly, as if I were cutting quickly with a scalpel. My tone of voice and Ginny's gentle hand were all we had for anesthesia.

"An average man with advanced lung cancer would not survive six months, but you have already proved you are not an average man. Not long ago you ran in the Marine Corps Marathon. You're tough."

His eyes reflected his mental activity as he absorbed my thoughts. He seemed to grasp the ray of hope I had given him while shaking off the threat of death, which clung like ballast to his heels.

He tried to mouth my words, but remained speechless.

I looked toward Ginny. Her head was in her hands. I felt a lump in my throat.

"I am saying life is possible, Toby. I'm saying we're in this together for the duration and there's no way I'm giving up on you. Calling in the hospice is just a way of getting help when we need it. I'll stick with you in this race until the finish!"

It was my last shot. I was drained of energy. If Toby lost hope, I would be unable to restore it. As I waited for his answer, deep inside I felt a visceral prayer reaching up to heaven.

He looked numb, as if he had not heard me, as if his mind had retreated to some safer realm than my somber talk provided. Slowly, as if a curtain were being drawn across his face, I saw a hint of a smile.

"It's like running the marathon," he said at last. "At fifty-two I was doing well just to enter, and I *finished*!"

"Right, Toby!" I said. "Against high odds you *finished*!"

"And you're saying I *could* live more than six months," he said. "I'm not going to let a signature on a scrap of paper change my life. I'm going to beat this damned thing. I'll be glad to have the hospice come to my house."

In our conversation, Toby had accepted the likelihood of death with the slim hope of survival. We had negotiated a victory in the setting of defeat. The victory had meaning for Toby. It meant I respected him and his values. It meant I would stick with him in the final stages of cancer without calling him a "treatment failure."

Agreement was possible because we shared common goals. We wanted to preserve his dignity and yet protect his family from undue suffering. For despite being a fierce competitor, Toby ranked his family's needs before his own.

10
SELF-ESTEEM

> I'm nobody! Who are you?
> Are you nobody, too?
> —Emily Dickinson

OUR self-esteem, our sense of dignity, our private evaluation of how we feel about ourselves and how we wish others to behave toward us constitutes a window of vulnerability when we have cancer. For whatever contributes to our sense of self-confidence, significance, power, capability, and independence, whatever makes us feel lovable and able to love, whatever enables us to adapt to the conditions in which we find ourselves, these all are threatened by the physical, emotional, and social changes that accompany the disease. A diagnosis of cancer exposes the most private parts of our bodies and our personalities to the blazing light of public evaluation. Issues we would have been free to decide for ourselves may be widely discussed, not only by professionals, but by family, friends, and journalists. We are transformed from casual randomness to statistically projected casualties, all by the stroke of the pen that wrote the word *cancer* beside our names.

If self-esteem were easily defined, it might be possible to make a general statement about the effect of cancer on our sense of self. But, whether healthy or ill, some of us have a clearer vision of ourselves than others. When asked to describe ourselves, some of us readily identify our physical attributes, family relationships, religious affiliations, public images, professions or occupations, titles or activities. Others have more difficulty finding a definition that suits them.

"I used to dance," one elderly woman told me, as if her life had ceased to have persistent shape or meaning in the decades that had passed since she last slipped into her pointe shoes.

Our image of ourselves *with* cancer is heavily influenced by our image of ourselves *without* it. If we have been satisfied with our daily lives, content with our relationships, supported by a network of affectionate family and friends, our experiences with cancer are likely to be vastly different from those of others who have been insecure and unfulfilled, divorcing or divorced, at odds with public institutions, engaged in lawsuits, and isolated. The latter are likely to bring with them fewer resources to cope with the assaults upon their dignity that caring people can provide.

Someone once told me that the best way to learn to cope with a fatal illness is to learn to live life well when you are healthy. Death may still be unwelcome when it comes, but you won't feel as cheated.

Cyril was bright, competent, and highly regarded by people who understood his abilities as an historian. He wrote great books in the privacy of his study and ventured into the outside world only to give lectures to academic audiences. On such occasions, he was meticulous in every aspect. He was always clean-shaven, dressed in a freshly pressed suit, and sporting a tie with regimental stripes. His public appearances sufficed to make him extremely popular among a wide group of enthusiastic history lovers, who regarded him as an inspirational leader. His response to their support was characteristically modest. When asked, he would have proclaimed that his wife, four children, and eight grandchildren were of utmost importance to him.

When Cyril developed cancer, he found that weakness and pain made it difficult for him to concentrate upon his work. Although he had spent his days writing, when the cancer grew, he was unable to write at all. Indeed, the energy required to shave and dress exhausted him, so that he found it far more practical to spend his days lounging, unshaven, in a robe, using his meager energy for the most essential tasks. He refused to talk about his cancer, hiding it from everyone but his wife. His secretiveness and seclusion were of such a marked degree that he was advised to take antidepressant medication or to see a psychiatrist. He asked me what I thought about it.

"This is a new role for you, Cyril, one for which you have not been prepared by previous experience or training. In the past you have excelled at research, writing, and lecturing. You have been an exemplary father. Your appearance has been faultless. Now you are challenged to find within yourself the capacity to refocus your energy on the issues of highest priority. I would guess that means your family. Have you been open with them?"

"I don't want them to see me. I look disheveled, like a bum. I'm surprised you even recognize me."

"Your physical appearance is not nearly as important as your presence."

"I hate to see the look of suffering in my family's eyes."

"But have you told them how you feel? Have you reminded them that your brain is still healthy even if your body has been attacked by a disease? Have you said that, while you can, you want to continue to function as a family, to talk about what is happening to you, to hear their feelings as they hear yours? This cancer you have, you did not choose to have. It is not your fault. You cannot relieve the pain your family feels by hiding from them. Hiding your feelings only feeds their fear."

We know better than to label people as cases of disease. Labels segregate people into "them" and "us." They hurt. The *language* of segregation is now considered unacceptable. But the *attitude* survives, conveyed by not-so-subtle phrases and hints of *otherness* when people who don't have cancer talk to people who do.

I believe the sense of *otherness* has done as much to undermine self-respect as the other problems caused by disease or treatment. Social isolation is more deeply felt because of the weariness caused by the symptoms of cancer and the heavy burden associated with dealing with the medical establishment, the treatments and complications, the disability and the fear of death. When added to the unavoidable burdens, the pain of social isolation can cause severe depression and lingering pain.

Such pain may be caused by well-meaning friends, caring but thoughtless people, who did not realize that pity adds to human misery. Such pain may be caused by unwelcome and unneeded advice. Such pain may come when people, instead of asking us, assume they know how we feel.

After a string of these assaults, is it any surprise when human relationships cease to make some people with cancer feel good? After a while, some of them may even cut off communication.

Before he got cancer, Toby had a high measure of self-esteem. On a scale of one to ten, he was a definite ten. He was a proud father, a devoted husband, an expert at what he did. As an exercise enthusiast, he had more than proved he could endure hours of preparation in order to compete with younger runners. He had a circle of friends who envied him his health and stamina. But cancer changed all that.

Toby's self-esteem stemmed from the things he did and cared about. Because he could no longer jog, Toby could not depend on this activity to replenish his enthusiasm for life. He found it difficult to talk about the things that made him feel important, powerful, or in control. Despite his strong interest in family, friends, athletics, and his consulting work, he rarely mentioned any of them.

"Just make me well, Doctor," were his constant words to me.

By "well" I knew he meant well enough to do the things he loved: to travel, to play with his grandchildren, to direct programs for his employer, and to run. He had lost the exhilaration that came from running, the sense of accomplishment that always came when he rounded the top of the hill on the homeward stretch, and something else that runners can't explain. As close as Toby and I became, because I was not a runner, I could not comprehend what it was he had lost. He told me about a mystical experience serious runners recognize, a defining moment which changes their lives forever.

"Forever?" I asked.

"From that point on," he said, "there is no finish line."

By his own declaration, Toby had been a serious runner for more than fifteen years before he got cancer. Fifteen years of running for his life, of finding a glowing, special, otherworld experience almost daily, wherever he was, at home, on the beach, in other countries, in marathons. And while the running lasted, there was no finish line. But the running had ceased. Forever.

After weeks of retraining, Toby bragged about walking from the front door to the curb. But his voice cracked when he told me about it, and I knew better than to applaud with too much enthusiasm. I was available, not to replace, but to substitute for his friends, the serious runners, who could, merely by making eye contact, let Toby know they understood his feelings. It was my responsibility to help him feel he was still in a race that counted, a race we must continue *as if there were no finish line,* even though we knew there would come a time when the race would end. Forever.

Toby and I recognized a certain chemistry in our relationship from the start. The strength of our relationship came from our ability to go beyond his cancer and what I could or could not do about it. I cared about Toby, and he about me. We endured our doctor–patient relationship out of grim necessity. We enjoyed each other as people.

I think one important bond that linked us was the satisfaction we both took in being able to give of ourselves to others. Rather than regarding the needs and expectations of our families as a burden, we felt grateful for the opportunity to gain significance by doing what we could for them. When Toby could give something to someone else, he thrived.

Weakness, shortness of breath, and occasional pain limited Toby's ability to act as he might otherwise have done. But even at a time when he rarely left the house except to come to my office, I discovered he had made a forty-mile trip by car with his daughter, Billie, the art history major who was "between jobs." When I asked the purpose of the trip, he told me it had helped him more than chemotherapy.

"What did you do?" I asked.

"I encouraged her to develop her skills in computer art," he told me. "She needed a printer. I helped her select one that would work best for her. She's an artist, you know," he added with a wink. "She's creative, but she doesn't know much about technical equipment."

Toby taught me something about the therapeutic value of allowing people with cancer to do things for the people they care about. When his daughters first came to visit me, I had told them to stay close to Toby and give him all the help they could. I had missed the mark. It was more important for Toby to help *them* as much as he could.

One of the more mystical of human qualities, the spirit of optimism, begs definition. Like a rare perfume, the sweet scent of optimism enhances the personalities of those who have it and lightens the hearts of other people whose lives they touch. If it could be distilled, purified, and given as a medicine, we would have a valuable elixir to remedy the pessimistic, the fearful, and the depressed, who seem to be more numerous than their happier counterparts.

I first met Drake a month after his wife died. They had been married fifty years. For most of their lives together, they had both enjoyed good health, but her health had failed nine years before she died. She had a major heart attack, and Drake retired from work in order to care for her. His love for her remained steady despite the years of nursing her.

"I loved her, and I would have gone on loving her," he said. "I cared for her day and night for nine years. That poor woman suffered so much; I would not have wanted her to endure another minute of it. It may sound heartless, but I'm glad it's over."

A month later, he returned for a physical examination, the first he had been able to have for almost a decade. He had no complaints. He felt strong and vibrant. He was seventy-three years old. When I examined his prostate, I found a hard nodule. I told him I suspected prostate cancer.

At my suggestion, Drake contacted a urologist. He appeared to have a limited cancer that could be cured with radiation therapy. He underwent the treatment, rarely complaining about the side effects. Two months later, I performed another rectal examination. The nodule had not disappeared. I brought him back to my office to talk about it.

"As I see it," he said, "I've got no choice. I've got to live with it."

And live with it he did. He worked as a volunteer at a local hospital for several days each week. He brought smiles into patients' rooms.

"I tell them I have cancer," he said. "They see I don't look so bad, and it calms them down. So many times people are afraid because they don't know whether they'll be able to get up and around and do things. They think I'm there to make them feel good, but I'm the one who gets the most satisfaction, Doctor."

Despite his happy outlook, blood tests showed his disease was progressing. We started hormone therapy. His prostate cancer appeared to be spreading to the soft tissues in his pelvis. For a while he had blood in his urine. When that cleared, he developed paralysis of a nerve in his leg, which created a foot drop. He discovered the problem while traveling in Turkey. His toe caught on a cobblestone, and he fell flat on his face. Thanks to the speed and efficiency of international flight, he was in my office two days later. With bandaged nose and bruises extending from his forehead to his chin, he looked grotesque. But there was no mistaking Drake's radiant smile.

"I'm glad the fall was *after* dinner, Doc," he said. "It was quite a meal."

I fitted him with a foot brace, and he continued to travel. He went to Michigan and Florida, to Oberammergau and Ireland. He traveled with friends and enjoyed himself. He sent me descriptions of his adventures on the backs of colorful postcards. He never mentioned any distress he may have felt during his travels.

He grew partially deaf. His leg began to swell. The blood tests for prostate cancer were one hundred times the normal value. A scan of his abdomen and pelvis showed massive nodules. We changed his hormone treatment.

He had to rise several times during the night. His bladder was obstructed and failed to empty when he urinated. Another hormone treatment produced better results. The swelling in his leg diminished, and he was able to sleep three hours at a time.

He traveled to Myrtle Beach, Jacksonville, and Sarasota. He collected stories about people and places. He told me how much fun he had. He received an award for volunteering for five hundred hours at the hospital in three years.

After five years of almost constant symptoms from his prostate cancer, he came to visit me one day. As always, I was glad to see him.

"I wish I could do more for you," I said.

"I'm grateful," Drake told me. "Since my wife died, I've had cancer for five years, but I'm alive. I've been around this beautiful country of ours, I've gone to Europe and the Middle East. I've seen the passion play. I've spent many precious holidays with my family.

"I've enjoyed every minute of it. I haven't spent one night in a hospital. I've lived, laughed, and loved. I've never lacked for human companionship. I have two lovely daughters and eight wonderful grandchildren who care about me. I'm grateful, Doctor. That's all I can say."

⊠

Being misunderstood destroys self-esteem faster than hair loss or vomiting, surgery or chronic pain. Too often, professionals assume the people who seek their help have predictable feelings, want "cure at any cost," "cannot face reality," and are too overcome by anxiety to reason clearly. Sometimes it is the doctors who simply haven't listened.

"I hate to dump the Bridgets on you, Dan," Dr. Clodman said. "Milton Bridget acts as if he didn't know he has cancer. His wife, Reba, doesn't get the facts straight either. She's emotional and reacts to information with hysterical shouting and crying. She has criticized my treatment plan. They don't seem to understand the hopelessness of the situation."

I expected a slow boil, if not a volcanic eruption, when the Bridgets came to my office. I've seen my share of emotional reactions to cancer. Fear does strange things to sensible people.

Milton Bridget shook hands warmly before he sat down. I recognized him. He had a wide reputation as a local musician. My pleasure at meeting a famous man was mixed with regret because I knew I could not cure him of his cancer.

Reba accompanied her husband into my conference room. Although concern and fatigue had grayed her cheeks, she carried herself with dignity. I could tell from her bearing she wanted me to listen to every word.

"You wouldn't believe what we've been through," she said.

I settled back in my chair, prepared for a distorted, angry view of Milton's medical care.

"They misled us at first," she said. "When they took out his colon cancer, they told us surgery had cured him. They lied to protect our feelings. They knew his cancer would grow back. His abdomen was full of it. How long did they think their lie would last?

"A year later, when the cancer regrew, they told me he had to have chemotherapy. They said he would die if he didn't get it. We were on our way to Florida, so we arranged to have the chemotherapy there. He got horribly sick. He had diarrhea ten or twenty times a day. He lost weight. He couldn't eat. He couldn't even stand up without fainting. He had to be admitted to the hospital for intravenous fluids.

"I called the doctor and asked if Milton had to keep taking the treatment. I told him about the reaction. The doctor accused me of trying to kill my husband by stopping the treatment."

She looked at me expectantly.

"But there is no cure for him," I said. "Didn't the doctor tell you that? There isn't even a remote chance."

"I want help, Doctor," Milton said. "If something will give me a little time or enable me to feel better, I am more willing to try it. But I don't want to be lied to any more. I want to understand the truth about these treatments. I may not be a doctor, but I can understand enough about medicine to know what's happening to me, what the treatments can reasonably do. I want to be told."

"First of all, Milton," I said, "although it hurts to talk about it, you are going to die from this cancer. I can't cure it, and neither can anyone else. What I can offer is a hope of softening the illness, of treating the complications, the pain, and the problems. The chemotherapy may help if we adjust the dose so it doesn't give you diarrhea. I don't advise chemotherapy if it makes you sick. I don't think you would be better off."

"I am glad you are not afraid to be honest," Milton said.

I suggested a limited trial of chemotherapy. If he improved, we would continue it. If his cancer was still growing after two months, we would stop it.

"I want you to call me to report every side effect," I said. "If the medication makes you sicker, I want to know about it. It's my job to help you feel better. There's nothing to be gained by suffering in silence."

For the next two months Milton took chemotherapy. I gave him treatments once a week. Although he showed little in the way of improvement, he rarely called to register complaints.

Milton's popularity made him recognizable in the waiting room, particularly among professional musicians. On one occasion I found him engaged in an animated conversation with two other patients. He was reminiscing about old times in the orchestra pits of the silent movie theaters.

"You look terrific!" I said, still encouraged by the enthusiasm Milton had demonstrated in the waiting room.

"I feel terrible," he told me. "But I don't feel comfortable talking about my complaints to anyone except you and Reba. I have no appetite. My weight has dropped another fifteen pounds. My abdomen hurts. I sleep poorly. I'm weak."

Milton's body had experienced the ravages of advanced cancer. His robust laughter in the waiting room concealed his weakness, but his gaunt cheeks hinted at the degree of malnutrition he had suffered.

"I tried the supplements you offered," he said. "I couldn't swallow them."

"But Milton," I said. "You looked so confident and strong out there. How did you manage it?"

"Show business," Milton said. "After all those years in the orchestra pit, I know how to put on a performance. I've made a crowd cheer when I had a fever of a hundred and two."

The chemotherapy failed to work, and we agreed to stop it. A few months later, Milton could no longer stand up. He could not eat or drink. Severe pain racked his body to the point where I urged him to take intravenous morphine for comfort. To make life easier for Milton and his wife, I admitted him to the hospital. It was obvious to all of us that he would die within a few days.

When I came to Milton's hospital room, he was asleep. As I examined the nurse's progress notes, I happened to catch a glimpse of the television by his bed. It was tuned to a broadcast about local entertainment. I was surprised to see Milton being interviewed. Transfixed, I watched as he proceeded to recall events about his life as a professional musician. It had been a good career, he told the interviewer, because it had permitted him to bring happiness into people's hearts. I was amazed at how well he looked.

"Perhaps they taped the program many months ago," I thought. "Perhaps they are airing it in his honor."

Milton stirred, and I saw he was awake.

"You look terrific," I said.

"I don't feel terrific," he told me with a groan.

"I meant on television. When did you make the tape? You never mentioned it to me."

"I made the tape two weeks ago. I didn't tell them I had cancer."

"Why not?"

"I didn't want to worry them. You know how it is, Doctor: 'The show must go on!' "

⊠

Augusta, body ever held erect, stiff upper lip, with crisp British accent despite two decades in the States, remarked upon the need for plain talk about cancer from ordinary people.

"It's not what the television shows would have you think, at all!" she said. "I've watched people with cancer being interviewed on television, but the people being interviewed are often celebrities. They treat the whole thing like a magnificent opportunity to sneak some publicity for themselves. I would rather turn them off. They don't seem to feel it the way the rest of us do. One said, 'I had to get back to work. I had a show to do,' as if there were nothing much to it. Another said, 'When I got cancer, I cried my eyes out!' Well, I jolly well didn't cry *my* eyes out. Wouldn't have done a bit of good. It would have made things worse. I thought about my family. We're all very close, you know. We care a lot about each other, and I didn't want to hurt them. Besides, I'd had a devil of a time convincing my doctor that what I felt in my breast *was* a cancer. He didn't want to believe me. So I had to call someone else. By the time I had the biopsy that proved that it was a cancer, I was grateful to have it out. I wasted no time in self-pity!

"People are always saying, 'Go to a support group!' as if that would solve all my problems. Maybe that helps them, but it wasn't what I wanted. I took care of everyone else's needs, just as I've always done. I have a loving husband and two very loving sons. They're grown, you know, but terribly close to Mummy just the same. They needed looking after just as much as I did. I could see the pain they were feeling, just by looking in their eyes. We never talked about it, of course, but I knew better than to worry them with it by 'letting it all out.' So I followed doctor's orders and took care of myself. I felt I was being perfectly logical.

"After my surgery, they sent an Anglican priest round to see me. A pleasant chap, but he took it all a bit hard. He was appalled to learn that I had not informed my family back in England. I mean, I'd thought of it but decided against it as being terribly upsetting for them. There was my mum, who's well past ninety and quite forgetful. It would have been a chore just getting the word through over the telephone. Better to wait, I thought. I'd be back at home in six months' time. I would have recovered from my surgery, and they could see with their own eyes that there was nothing wrong with me. But the priest wouldn't hear of it. He talked as if it were a moral outrage to keep my family in the dark. Then he told me how upset he had been when *his* mother was in hospital and no one let *him* know. I felt sorry for him, but what did that have to do with my mum and me?"

Augusta was always accompanied by her son, a middle-aged man named Elbert, who carried a loose-leaf notebook and recorded my every word. The pair were an exception to our practice. Although many women come to us alone for consultations, most come with their husbands or daughters, almost never with their sons. The sons who come are rarely as attentive to detail as Elbert. Other sons spend their time in the waiting room reading, giving the outward appearance of detachment. In contrast, Elbert was totally involved.

At first, I reacted to Elbert with suspicion. He seemed to be hovering too close, to be overprotective. I wondered whether his mother might do better without so much attention.

But Augusta's son was not what I supposed. Although he was a careful, meticulous note taker, he did not hover because of his own needs. He came because she insisted on it. It was his job to listen to the details, little items she feared she would forget if he did not record them. Those little items meant more to her than generalizations. After she left my office, she would review the conversation with him word by word.

I began to see Elbert as a caring, intelligent young man, not overprotective, just available. Because, in the framework of their family, he was doing what was expected.

"You can always tell when doctors care about their patients," Elbert said. "The minute you walk into the office, you can tell. If the receptionists are warm and friendly, if the nurses seem ready to help, then the doctors care."

Sometimes self-esteem nestles deep within a large family. Cal had ten children, and while he was able, none of the children ever accompanied him to the office. He had a wispy, waxed moustache that curled at the ends. Cal wore sport shirts and cowboy boots, and his waxed moustache proclaimed his freedom to be himself. Cal's language was full of foul expressions. No sentence was complete without a string of four-letter words. For Cal, a person wasn't "crazy," he was "buggier than dogshit"; he was never "perspiring heavily," he was "sweating like a whore in church." But the untroubled tone of his voice gave his speech a beguiling comedy that kept it from sounding offensive. I never saw him angry.

I heard about the children from Cal. He was proud of them. They were all different, some more accomplished than others, some dutiful, some defiant, some educated, some plodding along. Cal's wife had been a nurse. She was quite matter-of-fact about his cancer. No one needed to tell her that she would watch her husband die. The only question she ever asked was, "What can I do to help?"

Between visits to my office, Cal pursued his hobby of overhauling automobile engines in his basement. While his wife and I exchanged knowing glances, he insisted that he knew what he was doing. We worried about the effect of lifting heavy weights upon his weakened back. Cal worried about what he would do if he was forced to stop lifting heavy weights. Despite our concern, he managed to hold himself together with pain medication and brute determination for many years. But the time came when he could not climb the basement stairs. His back ached, his thighs were weak, and there was nothing more I could do to improve his endurance.

His family arranged a visit in my office. Although the youngest of his children was in her twenties, Cal remained the unassailable head of the family. He ruled because he was an old-fashioned father, a stern disciplinarian, a leader with keen vision, a master of rhetoric. He ruled because he loved them. He ruled because they let him.

I was surrounded by Cal's ten children. Neither Cal nor his wife were with them. Some were relaxed, others distressed. Some were serious questioners, others were withdrawn, disturbed by information, reluctant to hear me speak. But they had all come.

They made the purpose of their mission clear. They wanted me to confirm their belief that the cancer was about to take its toll. His most outspoken child wanted me to tell the others when Cal was going to die.

"How is it important?" I asked. "Your mother wants to care for him at home. She will stay with him as long as it takes."

"She will never be alone, Doctor. Although we all have jobs and families, one of us will always be with her. We'll bring in meals, shop, take care of the errands, mow the lawn. Most of all, we'll be there next to him so he can keep on telling us how to run our lives. Not that we can't take care of ourselves. But it's his way of showing that he cares about us."

We rambled over many subjects for more than an hour. Each of Cal's children had an opportunity to speak. They listened to each other with respect, giving ear to grief and joy with equal attention. Comforting without silencing. Laughing painlessly at family foibles. Never forgetting who they were or why they were in my office. At length the conversation came to a close.

"We have done all we could," I said. "Cal certainly has done all he could."

I've seen and talked to many families over the years, but it was a rarity to see so many children at one time. As different as his children were from each other, Cal had captured every heart.

When I paid my final visit a few months later, I was surprised to see that the house in which Cal had raised his large family was rather small. I wondered how they had raised so many happy children in such a modest house. Love, it would seem, makes the improbable possible.

"Doc's comin'," Cal told his wife before I arrived. "Better put some Scotch in the fridge. Don't want to insult the man."

He had lost weight; his hair was thin and grey; he could barely rise from bed. His face was wan, and he looked tired. But there was still a glint in his eye, and he looked like a rake in his silk pajamas with naked women on the lapels. And, sure enough, he was still sporting the neatly curled waxed moustache.

"They keep me warm at night," Cal told me, fingering his lapels. "About all I got left are dreams. My pecker ain't worth spit. Besides, those hormones made my tits so big I've got *men* asking for my phone number."

Antique furniture filled the tiny bedroom, giving it a homey air. Photographs of his family crowded the walls. I sat at his bedside while he described each scene, recalling the holidays with a twinkle in his eye. His wife brought tea and cookies. The three of us sat and talked about our families. I almost forgot that he was dying of cancer, that this would be our last visit.

"I'd like you to see a difficult patient," Dave told me.

Difficult patient is a you-know-what-I-mean kind of term without definition. Its imprecision offends me. *We doctors* are the ones with the difficulty. People don't plan to be patients the way we plan to be doctors. It just happens to them. As physicians, we have to take them the way they come. It may make our work harder sometimes, but no one ever promised us it was going to be easy.

Even though I did not care for the term *difficult patient*, I have a deep respect for Dave. A senior physician with years of clinical experience, he has an even temper and a gentle voice. When Dave said *difficult patient*, he meant he had tried to respond to his patient's demands and felt he had not accomplished much.

But it was worse than that. Minutes before Baruch arrived, Dave called me with a last-minute comment.

"I called his daughter," Dave said. "She told me Baruch had told her to drop dead."

When I ushered Baruch into my office, I became aware of the vastness of my task. Baruch had cancer, and he knew it. But he knew nothing about it. He did not understand how the cancer that now filled his liver could have started somewhere else. He did not understand why Dave had wanted to look for the tumor somewhere else or why, when he failed to find it, he had abandoned the search. The ideas would have been difficult to convey if he were calm, but he was not at all calm.

Aside from the confusing work of explaining the details of his diagnosis, I had to tell him what it meant. My years of experience had taught me that there was no cure for Baruch. Indeed, my best therapies would be worthless to him. The cancer filled his liver. He had lost at least thirty pounds. He was weak, short of breath, and fatigued. Blood tests showed his liver functioned poorly. As I ushered him into my office, he limped behind me.

"I'll make it," he said. "Just give me time. I need lots of time,

Doctor. I hope you're not one of those doctors who rush with their patients."

His face was the brown grey of a dusty road after a month with no rain. It had been several days since his last shave. His mouth drooped in perpetual sadness. His eyes had lost their luster. His abdomen protruded visibly as he sank into the armchair. I could see him heaving with every breath, as if he were chugging upstairs. His legs were swollen. He looked battered and worn out.

As I closed the door, I sensed the misery of a condition that added to his cancer. He was alone.

He had been alone in my waiting room and in my office. I soon learned that he was alone in his car and alone in his house. His wife had divorced him twenty-four years earlier. I knew nothing of the circumstances but surmised that they had been unpleasant. He mentioned that his ex-wife had convinced one of their daughters never to speak to her father after her eighteenth birthday. And she never did. He had one other daughter, the one he had told to drop dead, but she had married badly, suffered from abuse, and lived at a distance. Baruch's parents and siblings had long since died. He had been retired for ten years. He had few friends.

He was alone, and he was a stranger to me.

Before we talked about his cancer, I wanted to know him better. I discovered idle banter was not his style. He was an attorney. He had a list of questions on a legal pad and a brace of sharpened pencils. He wanted answers, not friendship.

So I listened to his questions, all of them good ones. Why does it hurt when I breathe? Why am I so short of breath? What can you do about the pain? Why have I lost weight? Is the swelling in my ankles serious? Why can't I get an erection? What kind of treatment are you going to use? What is the prognosis? Three months? Six months? What will my insurance cover? Will I be able to drive? What can I eat? What *should* I eat? Will vitamins help? Will alcohol hurt? Is there any hope at all? Why did I have all those barium studies? Do you need to do more tests?

Baruch and I had an hour or so to find each other. I wanted to answer as many of his questions as *he* could tolerate because he wanted to know. Why else the legal pad and so many pencils? But some were complex, some of grave consequence, some mysteries to me as well as to him. I pondered for a while, trying to decide where to begin. He helped me.

"I have never been more frightened by anything in my life. That includes the war," he said.

"Where did you serve?" I asked.

"ETO, '44 and '45," he replied.

"E . . . E . . . European?"

"European Theatre of Operations."

To me this suggested two possibilities. D-Day and Patton. I have known men who landed on Normandy beach and men who marched with Patton. Hoping I could find a path to understand more about Baruch, I asked about his role in the invasion. I was unprepared for his reply.

"Armored," he said.

"What does 'armored' mean?" I asked. Tanks, he explained. A wall of steel advancing towards the east. He rattled off some numbers to identify the division.

"Forty-five hundred in each flank, a thousand in reserve. We were the advance group. We broke up the economy, invaded the territory, softened up the resistance. When we were surrounded by the Krauts (this was 1991!), the troops would come in and rescue us. I survived, but I have had a hatred of anything that came out of Germany ever since. They all stink with their smug kissers sticking up in the air, pretending they had nothing to do with it! I don't want to talk about it."

No helpful memories to be had. No sentimental feelings about friends who died or a self-confidence begot by the courage he must have had or a philosophy of life resulting from his fortunate survival. Just hatred. I had *less* to work with than before I listened to his war experience, or so I thought.

"I want to look everything over before I answer your questions," I said. "Let me examine your body, the slides, talk it over with my colleagues."

"I understand," he replied, his lips hovering on the edge of a smile. But he asked several questions again, anyway. I worked on some of the simple ones.

"I can see you want to help me," he said. "I spent six years as a Federal inspector. It was my job to blow the whistle on bad doctors, slap them with prison sentences. There was some lousy, stinking stuff going on out there. 'Course all that was thirty years ago. Things have probably changed. New problems. New ways of cheating the system. But you and that other doctor, you seem to have the right idea. In fact, I hope you *are* like him. He's the finest doctor I have ever known."

I thanked him with a nod. In my awkwardness I feared that too much confidence could lead to excessive expectations. It would almost have been easier if Baruch had distrusted me. At least I would not have run the risk of disappointing him.

"About the prognosis," I said at a later date. "A lot of that depends on you. If you give up, you will not last long. If you make an effort to stay alive and if we look for the best treatment, you can maximize your life expectancy. None of us is going to get you out of here alive, but working together beats quitting. And if the enemy surrounds us, we'll call in the reserves."

A real smile this time.

"You are going to need help soon. What about your family?"

He told me his family had cut him off.

"Is there anyone else?" I asked.

"I have a friend," he said. "But I don't want to trouble her."

I settled back in my chair as he talked about his efforts to find a friend to ease his loneliness. He had wanted someone with whom he could share the quiet moments of his life. Someone who expected nothing more from him than simple caring.

"Knowing someone cares about you is the only thing that matters," he said.

Not the family, not the war experience, not the job that taught him to distrust physicians, but the glowing embers of a secret romance were the clue to Baruch's heart. I had found it, not by probing, but by caring about what happened to him.

"Was I too much of a son of a bitch?" he asked as we finished.

"I don't think so," I said.

"This may sound stupid," he said, lowering his gaze. "I know it's mid-November and, what the hell, I don't know how much time I've got. I have so many plans I'll have to give up. But," he paused to look at me, "I want to plant some daffodils."

"That doesn't sound stupid at all, Baruch."

11 DEATH

> The miserable have no other medicine
> But only hope.
> I've hope to live, and am prepared to die.
> —*Measure for Measure,* III, 1

I DO NOT believe death is evil. I think of it simply as biological fact. Death is as important a part of human life as birth.

The urge to survive is one of our strongest impulses, one that outlasts most others. Because death thwarts our will to live, we fight to avoid it. As a consequence, rather than give death due respect, we are inclined to regard it as a punishment. Instead of thanking our creator for not making our lives interminable, we act as if good people do not *deserve* to die.

We need death as much as food and water. Without death, living tissues could not repair themselves. Without death, new growth could not squeeze out old. If our ancestors had not died, we would have to settle for less of everything. If we do not die, the earth will be unlivable when our grandchildren's grandchildren arrive.

Although our lives end with death, our individual marks do not vanish. If the remnants of mindless life in the form of fossils, fuels, and rock remain a part of our world today, how much more will *our* lives persist through our children, inventions, art, construction, and archival collections. Only imagination limits our endurance.

While most of us do not welcome death, young people resist it mightily. Yet our capacity to use life well depends less on the number of years we live than it does on the choices we make. Short-lived individuals have made profound impressions. Vincent van Gogh produced most of his famous works during a span of less than four years. He died at thirty-seven, as did George Gershwin and Robert Burns. Mozart died at thirty-five, Alexander the Great at thirty-three, Schubert at thirty-one. Stephen Crane lived only twenty-nine years. Anne Frank, whose diary helped keep love alive in a world rocked by hate, was only a teenager. But Millard Fillmore, the Know-Nothings' candidate in 1856, lived to be seventy-four.

When life becomes unbearable, we appreciate the balm of death. Like Jonah, who wished for death simply because his gourd had perished, we sometimes long for death too easily. Happily, our bodies can outlast such fleeting thoughts. Yet it would be evil indeed if we were forced to live for more than a century, racked with pain, helpless and aware of our helplessness, draining the wellsprings of love from those we cared about, simply because we could not die.

People whose lives have been encumbered by miserable disease have learned to see death as a sweet deliverance. Their families have often found the end to be a blessing. Love and understanding helped them to accept what none of us can avoid.

As fervently as I believe the previous paragraphs, I had to force myself to write about Toby's death. People often say to me, "You must be *used to it* by now," but I don't think oncologists ever get used to it. Not if they care.

By early June, the end was near for Toby Thompson, and both of us knew it, even though we did not talk about it. I wanted him to be well enough to smile and to feel good about himself. I spurned the thought that death might be a balm for him, despite my awareness of its inevitability. His thoughts mirrored mine as he planned for a future that could never be more than a fantasy. Yet, painful as his death might have been for me, I felt a responsibility to record the events so others might understand.

Within a few days the hospice society had enveloped his house with loving attention. Nurses had provided him with oxygen, a mechanical bed, and the essentials that make home care comfortable. Both the nurses and Toby called me often. Even his daughter, Julie, who had taken leave from her job, had been pleased with the arrangements. A call came at ten o'clock one Friday.

"I can't breathe," Toby gasped into the telephone. "I've got to be admitted."

"I'll meet you in the emergency room," I said.

After I examined him, I did not think Toby's breathing was severely compromised. Indeed, his respiratory rate without oxygen was only moderately increased. I knew at once he would be able to go home, but I said nothing until after I examined him.

"What happened?" I asked.

"I don't know," he said. "I got up and walked to the bathroom. It was too much for me. I got scared. Maybe I need some intravenous diuretic."

"But the nurse gave you a diuretic at home."

"No, Doctor. She *tried* to give it to me, but I stopped her. I wanted to have it here, where you could watch me."

"He feels so much safer with you watching him," his wife said gently. She was standing a few feet behind.

Silently, I wondered why. The hospice nurse had been present at every crisis. She had listened to his complaints, examined his lungs, prescribed accurately. She had called me before treating him to be certain we were in agreement. I thought she had given him better care than I could because of her availability and her willingness to visit his home on a daily basis.

"The hospice nurse has been very good to you," I said.

"She's wonderful," they said in unison. "But Toby has known you longer."

I gave Toby another dose of intravenous diuretic. His chest X-ray showed no evidence of fluid, and although his lungs gurgled a bit, I doubted much fluid had accumulated. I could not know for certain, but I thought cancer accounted for most of his problems.

"When am I going to receive more chemotherapy?" Toby asked. "You don't talk about that any more."

"You had two courses of it," I said. "It didn't help. I'm reluctant to continue. I know it will make you sick. I don't think it will shrink the cancer much at this point."

He looked disappointed but not surprised. I smothered my sense of defeat. Despite our agreement to accept the probability of death, I still felt the urge to tip the scales in his favor, to help him escape from an illness that held him in its claws. Yet the physician in me forced me to concentrate on *his* needs rather than my own.

"I'd like to send you home," I said. He nodded assent.

I left the city for a few days; when I returned, I found a message waiting for me: "Toby wants to be admitted." I called the house. I discussed the situation with Toby and his wife. His care at home had been almost ideal. The nurse had provided him with diuretic and morphine. She had visited him twice daily, even on the weekend. He was surrounded by friends and family. He lacked nothing, yet he wanted to be in the hospital.

"What can I give you in the hospital that you can't get at home?" I asked.

"Please, Doctor, I beg of you. This isn't working."

"I'm not going to refuse you, Toby. I just want to understand."

I yielded to Toby's wishes, still uncertain of his need. A distinct change had occurred. Although he claimed to be eating well, the hollows in his temples signaled his loss of muscle mass. His lips were drawn back, and his teeth were dry and sticky.

"They were all there," he said.

"Who?" I asked.

"My family," he panted.

"He asked them to come," Ginny said.

Wordlessly, Toby had come to terms with his condition. The

telephone had not sufficed for the messages he wished to impart.

"He tried to be his old self," Ginny said. "He laughed and chatted with them. He acted like nothing much was happening."

"I did not want to worry them," he said.

"The kids kept running around the house. The relatives needed to be fed. We were in the middle of constant commotion."

"It was too much for you," I said, hoping to strike a resonant chord.

"It was too much for her," Toby said, pointing a bony finger at his wife.

Ginny grinned sheepishly. His daughter, Annie, showed me a chart on which she had written in large blocks the time of day and the name and dose of each medication Toby was to take. A glance made it apparent that, although I had thought his regimen was simple, it was much too complicated for Ginny to follow.

"Besides," Annie added, "her vision is worse at night. She was afraid she might make a mistake in his medications and cause him serious harm."

I examined Toby. His resting respiratory rate was three times normal despite the oxygen flowing into his nose. The breath sounds were louder and more labored.

"It's like jogging on a hot day," I said. "You need a rest."

"I get tired when I try to chew or swallow," Toby said. "I can't eat solids, and I can't take big sips of liquids."

I felt as if I could see the finish line. Unless Toby's breathing slowed, the muscular effort would exhaust his energy reserves.

"We're going to use a morphine drip," I said.

"What's that?" Toby asked, looking worried. "I don't want to be a junkie."

"Addiction will not be a problem," I said. "We will be using the medication to slow your respirations and relieve the anxiety and pain of breathing. The two of us will control the morphine so you will be awake and able to communicate comfortably without feeling so desperately short of breath."

"Are you certain it will be safe?" he asked.

"I haven't the slightest doubt. Even if we miscalculate and give you a little too much morphine, the effects can be rapidly reversed with an intravenous antidote. Morphine is one of the safest drugs I know."

In the hall a cluster of women waited for me. His sisters, aunts, and others had flown in from New York and California. They looked at me expectantly with cheery faces, as if they hoped for a favorable report. Their smiles made me hesitate.

How could I welcome them when all I could think about was my gloomy message? I felt certain Toby had less than two weeks to live. Wouldn't his relatives, who but a short time ago had been laughing at his bedside, be bitterly disappointed to learn this reunion would be their last?

"So you were there when Toby got pneumonia sixty years ago," I said. Several acknowledged they had been. A minor dispute arose as to which of them had actually stood vigil with his long-since departed mother and which of them had only heard the much-repeated story of Toby's remarkable recovery afterwards. Finally, one of Toby's aunts clarified it.

"I should know," she said. "I am Toby's oldest aunt. I was like a mother to all of them."

"You remember when Toby's mother carried him to the Church of Our Lady of Mt. Carmel?"

"How could I forget? She was so grateful, she went barefoot through the center of Manhattan. Of course, you couldn't do it now. But she thanked God for Toby's life with her last breath."

"It was a wonderful story," I said. "And Toby has had a good life with success in every way, with children and grandchildren, professional recognition . . ."

"Excuse me, Doctor," the elderly aunt asked, "but are you trying to tell us Toby is dying?"

"I guess so," I said.

"Well, get on with it, then," she said. "You haven't got all day. You have other patients who need you, too."

With the aid of a diagram, I explained the breathing problem to them. Each watched with interest as I showed the relationship between the number of calories he was able to consume and the number he burned with the work of breathing.

"Thank you for being honest with us, Doctor," the ladies said. "We wanted to know."

"But I have to add something that you may not want to hear," I said. "Toby has little energy, and the work of visiting with you has exhausted him. In order to make it possible for him to save his strength, I have put a sign on his door excluding all visitors except for Ginny and their children. It is better for you to return home."

No one murmured. Although his sister had seemed on the verge of tears when I told her Toby was exhausted, she, too, nodded assent.

"We understand," they said, as if speaking with a single voice.

I believed them.

For the remainder of his life, I visited Toby every day. Rather than the hasty hello, which was all his medical supervision required, I sat at his bedside and gave him as much time as I gave my other patients. By then I was sure his breathing difficulties were solely due to cancer and further removal of fluid would be useless. I continued to give him oxygen. I monitored his breathing with a stethoscope. Each day I inquired about pain and anxiety, bowels and bladder, diet and energy. Together we catalogued the problems. Together we made plans to adjust his regimen in response to them.

During the following week I noticed a subtle change in Toby's conversation. For months Toby had talked about a range of subjects. His focus shifted to his bodily functions. He obsessed about little details, like clipping his nails, the placement of his urinal, the timing of his bath. He complained of sleeplessness and noxious dreams.

"It's all a big puzzle," he said, one morning.

"What's a big puzzle?" I asked.

"I don't know. Life, I guess. It's like a big computer program, the biggest one I've ever done, and there's a puzzle in the middle of it, and when I solve the puzzle, it will come."

"What will come, Toby?"

"The big one," he said. "Death."

"Do you want to talk about it?"

"No," he said, smiling impishly. "I have to save my strength to breathe."

Two mornings later, he was shaved and smiling when I arrived. His grasp was firm when I shook his hand.

"I'm going to get out of this place," he said. "I'm not giving in to this damned cancer. I'm going home where I belong."

"Today?" I asked.

"When I get my strength back. I'll need a little more time yet."

His second wind lasted only a few hours. By mid-afternoon when I checked back, he was too weak to talk much. Although Ginny told me he was still eating well, the hollows in his temples had deepened during the previous six days. Despite eating, his body was not deriving much nourishment from the process.

Together we adjusted the morphine drip to relieve his pain and the distress of rapid breathing. After two or three days he felt more comfortable. Several telephone calls were required. Although this meant repeated interruptions of my office schedule, it was important to ease Toby's distress. During each conversation I asked the nurse to count his respirations and to ask him how he felt before I adjusted the dosage of the morphine.

Ginny was ready for Toby to die before I was. She told me she had agreed to have him admitted to the hospital, expecting his life would soon be over. She never questioned any of my decisions, but she urged me to keep him out of pain.

"What will it be like?" she asked.

"A gentle sleep," I said hopefully.

As the last week of Toby's life began, I felt somewhat sullen, more sensitive to criticism, unable to laugh, even at funny jokes. I found it almost impossible to keep from thinking about Toby.

I continued to force myself to sit beside his bed once a day. Reluctantly, I dragged a chair from the corner in order to be closer to him. At times I felt more like a grieving visitor than a doctor. I could have provided adequate technical care by reviewing his orders with the nurse. But there was another purpose for my visits. I had become an important person in Toby's life, someone who could listen to what was churning inside his head. He wanted me to know, and it was my duty to listen. One morning I sat beside his bed waiting for him to speak. For a long while he said nothing.

"It wasn't so great," he said.

I strained to catch the syllables. His voice was faint, and it seemed as if something sticky was caked in his throat.

"What wasn't so great, Toby?"

"My sleep. Every time I fell asleep, I woke with a jerk. We can't have that."

"Does it hurt?"

"No. I don't hurt anywhere."

"Do you want more morphine?" I asked.

"I guess."

Several times as I watched, he drifted into a doze. His eyes were half open, but he seemed to be miles away. I wondered if he would die while I sat there, and yet each time I thought perhaps he was about to find permanent rest, he would open his eyes and begin to talk as if he had been awake all the time. His words sounded rational despite their irrelevance to his physical condition.

"I know now we have no control over it."

"Over what, Toby?"

"Over death. It comes when it comes."

I nodded, afraid my voice might not sound as calm as his.

"And yet," he continued, "I still want more time. I don't know how much, but I want more."

"Perhaps it would be better to think about things you would like to do, rather than the amount of time. What would you like to do?"

He was quiet for a while. He drifted into sleep for a few minutes. I thought he might have missed my question. I was prepared to let it go. I had asked in order to help him express his thoughts, to discharge some of the energy that had kept him alive for ten more days after we had thought he would die. I wanted to help him find peace.

"I want to travel with Pipsy," he said. "There are places we haven't seen."

"Who is Pipsy?" I asked.

"My wife. It's her nickname," he said. He flashed a grin. "I thought you knew."

"Oh, mind of man!" I thought. "There you are, lying in bed, weak as a kitten, within a hair's breadth of eternal rest, and you dream of travel with your wife as if it were a real possibility." But I listened as if I were discussing a wish list with a guest on a television talk show.

"I also want to see my next grandchild."

"When is the baby due?"

"In August," he said.

"But it's only June," I thought to myself. "I can't believe you have more than a few days left to live. Is it possible you'll prove me wrong?"

"You can always hope," I said aloud.

"It's going to be a girl," he said with a cocky grin.

"How do you know?"

"They did a sonogram, Doctor! It takes the mystery out of it, but it's more fun picking names."

"Two more months," I said.

"And then there's the christening in September," he said. "They're going to bring the baby up here so I can be a part of it."

He closed his eyes again. On tiptoe I returned the chair to the corner before I headed for the door.

"Maybe October," he called after me.

"Good-bye, Toby," I said, pausing at the door. "I'll see you tomorrow."

Seated at the nursing station, I called his wife. I described the conversation to her.

"Maybe it's for the best," I said. "Maybe it will be easier for him to go out still wanting to do things that he will never accomplish rather than admit the nearness of death."

The mental health nurse met me in the hall. She told me Ginny had been praying that each day would be his last. Ginny and Toby had discussed death openly many times. His fear of death had not prevented him from attending to practical necessities. He had made specific plans for his funeral. He had advised her about their house. He had given her a list of financial instructions.

We escalated the dose of morphine throughout the day. Towards evening the nurse called.

"He has a fever," she said. "His temperature is one hundred one."

"Is he in distress?" I asked.

"His family is concerned. Perhaps we should give him a rectal suppository. He can't swallow."

"I don't think he's going to live much longer."

"But Mrs. Thompson is upset."

I asked the nurse to bring Ginny to the telephone. I saw no value in medicating Toby for a fever.

"This is much worse than I thought," Ginny said. She let me hear her weep for the first time since our discussion in the intensive care unit six months earlier.

"What's wrong?" I asked.

"The croaking sound," she said, quickly regaining control of her trembling voice.

"The death rattle," I explained. "It doesn't hurt the person who is dying, although it may be painful for you to hear. He's in a coma, too deep to cough. He won't live more than another twenty-four hours now. Perhaps you would be more comfortable in the lounge than at his bedside."

"Maybe he can hear me," she said. "I want him to know we are nearby."

When I called an hour later, the fever had broken, and the breath sounds had become much gentler. Ginny had fallen asleep in the easy chair at the end of his bed.

"She was knitting a little pink sweater," the nurse told me.

Without knowing why, I awoke in the middle of the night. Inches from my face was an illuminated digital clock. The numerals flashed 3:40. I watched them for several seconds.

"Something's happened," I thought to myself.

The telephone rang with its all-too-familiar buzzing sound. The answering service informed me the Cancer Center had called.

"Mr. Thompson died," a nurse informed me. "His wife wants to speak with you. They want an autopsy."

I sensed a hint of disbelief in the nurse's voice. Very few families request autopsies.

"Hi, Dan," Ginny said. She sounded relieved. "Toby's troubles are over."

"Was it quiet?"

"For the most part. Whenever he complained of pain, the nurse gave him morphine, and he went right back to sleep. Julie and I asked for an autopsy. We thought it might help other people with cancer of the lung."

In death as in life, Toby and Ginny never missed an opportunity to show kindness to others.

"You have been wonderful to be so strong," I said. "Toby could always depend on you."

"Please come to the funeral service," she said.

Robert Frost wrote a poem entitled " 'Out, Out—' " about a young man who died. As if our significance on earth ended with death, he finished the poem as follows:

> No one believed. They listened at his heart.
> Little—less—nothing!—and that ended it.
> No more to build on there. And they, since they
> Were not the one dead, turned to their affairs.

Is that all there is? Is our quest for significance, which dominates so much of our thinking, limited by *mere* survival? There is a thought to justify terror of mortality.

When Hamlet mused about the "sleep of death," he never considered that he might be totally forgotten when he died. Shakespeare saved him from oblivion. Hamlet's body may have gone the way of Yorick's, but Hamlet will endure "so long as men can breathe or eyes can see."*

When Toby died, an emptiness sat upon my heart. As long as he struggled to cling to life, I had maintained my bond with him. With his death came a new challenge. I had to let go of what had perished and cling to what I could preserve. I had to grieve at the loss of a living being and console myself with the enduring memory of his friendship.

I went to the funeral in a state of unreality. The rituals of death as practiced at the funeral home declared a grim state of separation from which there could be no appeal. His smile, the glint in his eye, the squeeze of his hand, the sweat that coated his body after a long run, all the human forces that constituted his living energy had been forever laid to rest.

As much as I regretted being inside the mortuary, I was grateful to have a cool retreat from the torpid heat of early summer. I didn't much care for the solemn-faced attendants and the dull decor that greeted me, but I felt as if I belonged with the crowd of people ("Thompson's on the left, sir; O'Reilly's on the right.") who had come to pay their last respects. Indeed, I found some comfort in being included in Toby's funeral.

People sometimes ask me why I go to funerals. I often don't. When I do, I usually find it provides me an opportunity to affirm life as well as death. In taking leave of a person I cared about, I recognize the need to preserve the social bonds which were important to us both. Death would not be sorrowful if life were not of enormous significance. Binding myself with Toby's family and friends in the funeral home made me into something other than a mere cancer doctor. I was a part of the community which survived him.

Toby Jr. greeted me at the door. He spoke in hushed tones. I struggled to catch the words. His dark eyes reminded me of his father, but he seemed taller than I remembered. He remained in the antechamber. Further inside, I met Toby's sisters from New

*William Shakespeare, Sonnet 18, "Shall I compare thee to a summer's day?"

York and his aunt from California. They had spent a lot of time in airplanes in the previous two weeks.

Ginny kissed me, but I was unable to speak.

"I was there when he died," Julie told me. "It is the most significant thing I have ever done. I found I could soothe him by speaking softly and holding his hand. Most of the time he did not seem to understand what I was saying, but he knew I was there, and that was enough."

Perhaps Julie aroused some distant memory of Toby's mother, praying at his bedside when he was a tiny child. Had she inherited the timbre of her grandmother's voice, the gentleness of her touch?

Grieving at the finality of separation, I found immense comfort in Julie's words.

"He had some custard that evening, you know," Ginny told me. "He wanted to gain enough strength to leave the hospital. We can be glad he found a painless way out."

Later, I wrote a note to Ginny. In it I mentioned my feeling for Toby, his zest for life, his concern for his family, his sense of humor, and his willingness to fight to the finish.

I fight for life against almost certain odds. I fight because *they* fight. "They" are people with cancer, fellow humans caught in the grips of frightening illness, people who have been "given the message" by their doctors.

"My doctor painted a bleak picture," Sylvia said. "He made certain I understood I might die. He wasn't so clear about whether there was any chance I might live."

"Let us whisper the word *die*, Sylvia," I said. "Let us shout the word *live*. We have no need to be "clearly" told about horrors we can imagine only too well. A hint is enough to make us remember them all our lives. We all know cancer can be fatal. When a doctor says you have cancer, you get the message quickly enough."

"Have you been a patient?" she asked, laughing at my oration.

"I am as much a patient as you are," I said with a grin. "We are all people and only incidentally someone's patient."

Being an oncologist takes time and motivation. I must be willing to sit, to wait for permission to speak, to deliver information at a comfortable speed, to emphasize what is important without abolishing hope, to allay undue anxiety, to resolve confusion. It takes creativity and flexibility, written notes, drawings, graphs, and charts. It takes love and laughter, hugs and handshakes. Without them, the messages are bizarre distortions of what I meant to say.

"It sounds exhausting," Sylvia said.

"It doesn't feel that way to me. It feels like practicing the art of medicine. It feels right."

"When you said I had a chance, it opened a door for me," Sylvia said. "I felt as if I could breathe again. There is a world of difference between *almost* certain death and certain death."

"Of course, you understand there are serious risks and the treatment probably won't work," I said, after I had taken time to reassure her we would do our best to administer the medications carefully and to avoid any unnecessary pain or suffering.

"I do indeed," she said. "You described unpleasant possibilities, but there's also the possibility I might live. It's going to be hell, but there's still some hope."

❖

Not long after Toby's death, I was called to the viewing of a young woman named Joy. Although I did not have any desire to view her body, I felt I should respond to the call. Someone wanted me there.

I had just entered the hall of the funeral home when Joy's husband, Bill, met me at the door. I could see a throng of people huddled in the viewing room. I knew Joy was young, energetic, and eager to live. Surely most of the people in the room had closer ties to Bill and Joy than I did. Yet as I approached, insecure amongst a crowd of strangers, Bill hurried to me.

I would not have recognized him. His face was swollen, his eyes were bloodshot. He looked aged, weary. In fact, although I had seen Joy nearly once a month, I had not seen Bill in over four years.

He drew me into the nook of a nearby stairwell. I had my back to the crowd of mourners, but his gestures, his shaking frame, his anguished face were clearly visible to them. In our little enclave we were as private as if we had met in a crowd of strangers.

He wanted to tell me every bitter detail of her death. The details were painful for me to hear, far too painful to record. I found myself near tears as I listened. "Am I his doctor or his friend?" I wondered as I listened, of two minds whether I should "act professional" or vent my feelings.

I wondered why Bill had drawn me to this place, why he had selected me to hear memories that must have distressed him greatly. I had been drawn by a message left with my receptionist. Her name, the funeral home, and "viewing, 7 to 9, please come." I could easily have ignored the call. My family had just arrived from out of town. Dinner was waiting on the table. Yet before sitting down to eat, I had rushed to answer a call to view a body I did not want to see.

Memories of Joy when I first met her flooded my brain. Crisp and full of youth, she was a buoyant twenty-eight-year-old who did not look as if she had ever been pregnant yet had borne four children. During the fourth pregnancy, shortly before Christmas, she was found to have chronic myelogenous leukemia.

This form of leukemia, fortunately rare, has been doggedly persistent. While other leukemias have responded to treatment, this one kills with the same slow regularity common to its victims decades ago. For years the leukemia causes no symptoms; then suddenly it takes a sudden swing into a relentlessly aggressive phase. There are few survivors.

Her will to live prompted me to refer Joy to a physician who was committed to the task of finding a cure for chronic myelogenous leukemia. Cautious yet determined, he had tested many different forms of treatment without success. Indeed, in search of a cure, he had tested extremely toxic treatments with the unfortunate result that some of his patients had died from treatment rather than from the leukemia.

Joy had listened to his strategies and decided to continue milder treatment with me as long as she could. She remained stable for five or six years. One December she began to feel severe fatigue. Her blood tests confirmed her suspicion. The fatal phase was not far off.

With Christmas behind her, she returned to the medical center and was told about an experimental treatment. Preliminary results had been promising. She asked me whether she should try it.

"It's a long shot," I said, "but your options are limited. You'll have to make the decision."

She decided to take the experimental treatment. I have heard people compare cancer care to a roller coaster ride. I've ridden a few roller coasters. They're tame compared to the harrowing experiences of people with malignant diseases, who must confront difficult decisions and perilous treatments. No one hawks cotton candy after the ride.

"She seemed to do so well," Bill said. "Then all hell broke loose."

I listened while he told me the story of her final weeks in the hospital. Because I could think of nothing sensible to say, I remained silent.

Afterwards, he told me how well Joy had handled her illness in the early years. In six months, he told me, she had learned to cope with the leukemia. She had decided to get on with her life, to be a mother to her children, to return to work. He was the one who had faltered, he said, not Joy. While she had been learning to cope, he had become an alcoholic.

"She was doing well, and I was falling apart," he said.

I must have looked shocked. The leukemia had taken a double toll.

"Not any more," he said. "I don't drink now. It's a sickness I can conquer. Besides, the kids need me. They're great kids. Joy did everything she could to give them the strength to survive her death."

He sobbed. I took a deep breath, but my emotions overflowed. I put my arms around him and buried my face in his shoulder.

Perhaps he thought I was trying to comfort him, but in our little enclave underneath the stairs, more than one grown man needed a hug.

Soon afterward, at the end of a conference, I sought out the doctor who had tried to cure Joy's leukemia. It had been a long evening, but we were among the last to go. As we pushed our chairs under the table, our eyes met, and I could sense the sadness in his heart. For thirty years he had searched for a way of curing chronic myelogenous leukemia. Nothing had ever worked. His latest effort had been no better than the others.

"Keep trying," I said. "They're depending on you."

"It was terrible," he said.

"But Joy knew it could happen. We have to take risks in order to make progress. Risks are painful. Sometimes we lose. But it is better to die with hope than without it. You gave her reason to hope. I know she was grateful."

Months after Toby died, Ginny came to my office for a visit. Before we started our discussion, Ginny handed me a few sheets of paper. One contained a poem Toby had written about the deep significance of exercise. The other was a eulogy written by one of Toby's closest friends. It described him as a caring and competent individual, a man I would have valued as a friend during his years of health.

I had asked Ginny to come during the lunch hour so we might have a chance to talk with more leisure than the rest of the day afforded. I chewed on a sandwich while we spoke.

"The autopsy showed no surprises," I said. "Toby died of cancer. His lung was almost solidly replaced with it. I don't think any of our treatments ever helped him for more than a few weeks."

"At least you tried, Dan," she said. Her tones were even, almost unemotional.

"We did everything we reasonably could," I said. "Success was unlikely from the start, no matter how much effort we put into it. All I can promise is to provide the best known treatments, to pay attention to detail, to give people a chance to heal. I can't make it happen."

"But there was something much more important, Dan," Ginny said. "Something I don't understand too well."

"What's that?"

"He thrived on your attention. He doted on your words. Yet you never knew the man I married. Cancer changed him so much I scarcely recognized him."

I munched on a cookie for a moment, lost in thought.

"I believe you," I said. "Faced with severe illness, people undergo changes in their personalities. Our viewpoints alter; our priorities shift; we substitute new relationships for older ones. Our doctors, strangers until quite recently, suddenly become key figures in our lives. We bond to them like parents. Their words and gestures dominate our thoughts, their power over us seems almost boundless.

"I never know my patients as they were when they were well," I said. "I try to be aware of what is happening in their world in order to help them. But I am not a part of that world. In fact, if I become too much a part of their world, I lose my objectivity. I try to maintain a delicate balance."

"Toby was like you," Ginny said. "He made friends easily, let them feel they knew him. Yet most of the people he knew were not as close to him as they thought."

"I make myself available," I said. "I respond to questions, return telephone calls, deal with every issue, even issues unrelated to cancer. I listen."

"You do more than listen," Ginny said. "You're involved. You care about the outcome." She smiled.

Memories flip through my mind like pages in an old photo album, recollections of conversations with survivors. A nurse depressed at Christmas time, not because she had to work, but because her child had died. A doctor whose only child had died in an automobile accident. A woman in a department store whose husband had committed suicide. A friend whose baby had died at home. All I had done was to listen to them.

I am not alone. Many of us provide an audience for people in pain.

A patient who delivers "meals on wheels" believes that listening to the people who receive the food provides as much nourishment as the food itself.

A physician in practice believes good listening skills have provided greater benefits with fewer harmful side effects than any medicine he has ever used.

A former surgeon-general believes that devoting attention to teaching medical students how to listen may improve the relationship between the sick and the physicians who care for them.

A woman told me about a trans–Pacific Ocean flight during which the young man next to her described, in great detail, his concerns about his fiancée, a young woman with acute leukemia. The young man never asked the woman about her life. He would have discovered that cancer had taken the lives of her sister, her daughter, and two husbands. In addition, she had cancer herself. "He needed someone to talk to," she told me. "I was glad to be available."

Must we be in pain ourselves in order to understand people in pain? Must we have cancer before we can understand people with cancer? Or can we, because of our respect for human life, respond to people in pain or people with cancer by interrupting our own plans, by accepting our own mortality, and by taking time to listen?

AFTERWORD

A Time to Hear, A Time to Help began as the personal odyssey of a doctor who was motivated by an urge to express twenty-five years of emotionally charged experiences for which spoken words often seemed inadequate.

In writing this book, I reached toward others who shared my interest in listening to people with severe disease. As I collected material I learned a great deal about listening to people in distress, not from professors of medicine or other academicians, but from people with cancer and people in pain. The lesson is universal. The most sensitive barometers for measuring human suffering are our ears.

As I learned, I sought ways of improving my professional skills. I came to regard the art of professional listening as more than a descriptive device. It is my most cherished diagnostic and therapeutic tool.

In this Afterword I would like to identify books, writers, and teachers who influenced my work. I am deeply indebted to them.

I devoted a year to the study of the Book of Job with Rabbi Harold White of Georgetown University. The Book of Job is an ancient reaction to mutilating illness. Despite being layered with a Hellenic prologue and epilogue, its basic premise remains intact: God does not shield us from disaster.

The Book of Job is an excellent depiction of the emotional needs associated with critical illness and the limitations of comforters who refuse to listen to the sufferer. Repeatedly, Job's friends failed in their attempt to substitute their wisdom for his. Recurrently, he complained that they didn't have his story straight. Their arguments ended in an impasse.

A man named Elihu, one of Job's younger relatives, then delivered a monologue. He was long-winded, elaborate, and critical both of Job and his so-called comforters. Scholars and theologians have debated its place in the story, particularly because it was written at a later period than the rest of the book and Job never answered Elihu as he did his friends. But the monologue clearly shows the unwelcome intrusion of a self-righteous onlooker who volunteered his wisdom.

Only God, the One who always listens, gave Job an answer he could accept: human suffering is a part of human life, not a punishment by God. Fairness and justice are never an issue. No matter how righteous our behavior, God cannot interfere with the complex interactions of the universe to protect us from harm.

Job's story is timeless, as apt today as in the Biblical era. Thus, many authors have been prompted to write commentaries about it. Nahum N. Glatzer compiled over thirty of them in a book entitled *The Dimensions of Job.*[1]

I also studied Tolstoi's "The Death of Ivan Ilych,"[2] a modern classic about a man with cancer. Set in the middle-class society of late nineteenth-century Russia, the details have the richness of Tolstoi's other work. But because he concentrated on the experience of illness rather than the setting in which it occurred, segments of the story apply to people in our own time with very little alteration.

[1]Nahum N. Glatzer, *The Dimensions of Job* (New York: Shocken Books, 1969).

[2]Leo Tolstoi, "The Death of Ivan Ilych," in *The Death of Ivan Ilych and Other Stories*, translated by Aylmer Maude (New York: New American Library, 1960).

As an example, Tolstoy noted that Ilych's wife developed an

> attitude towards him and his disease . . . that he was not doing something he ought to do and was himself to blame, and that she reproached him lovingly for this . . . and she could not now change that attitude.

"You see he doesn't listen to me," Ilych's wife complained. No one, neither wife nor friends, *listened* to Ivan Ilych. Indeed, even the doctor paid little attention to him. When Ilych complained, "The pain never leaves me," the doctor responded, "Yes, you sick people are always like that," more concerned about warming up his hands than attending to his patient's pain. It is small wonder that this story continues to be a vital part of the education of anyone who would want to learn about the process of caring for people with cancer.

I was educated at the University of Chicago, in the same setting where Elisabeth Kuebler-Ross made her seminal observations on people with terminal illness, and I have always had a strong interest in the personal needs of people with cancer. When *On Death and Dying*[3] appeared, I was delighted at the prospect that hospital-based physicians might develop a more caring attitude toward fatal illness. Kuebler-Ross made no bones about her observations. Hospital-based American doctors regarded death as evidence of personal failure.

To help physicians cope with their insecurity in confronting dying patients, Kuebler-Ross devised a simplified system for analyzing human reactions, the now well-known "stages" of denial, anger, bargaining, depression, and acceptance. Her work helped many recognize certain behaviors as a by-product of coping with severe emotional distress, but the rigid format and the implied orderliness of progression from one stage to the next did not satisfy the professional needs of the medical establishment. Nevertheless, her work gave impetus to the hospice movement and led to the

[3]Elisabeth Kuebler-Ross, *On Death and Dying* (New York: Macmillan, 1969).

development of a disciplined approach to caring for people who are destined to die.[4]

Although *On Death and Dying* attracted attention to the needs of people who were near death, it did not respond to the needs of people who had cancer but were not dying. Indeed, the work in this field has not been commensurate with the astounding technical improvements in cancer care. Even today, some physicians are sufficiently awkward in discussing cancer with their patients that visits to doctors are traumatizing events.

The inadequacies of physicians are most apparent to us when we ourselves become ill. Besides my family members, many of my physician-friends have been troubled by cancer. Indeed, one of my classmates committed suicide shortly after her physician-husband died of lymphoma. Our system had not coped with her emotional needs.

A few years after receiving his degree, Dr. Fitzhugh Mullan, also a graduate of the University of Chicago, developed a rare tumor in his chest. Turning his personal tragedy into an opportunity for self-expression, Dr. Mullan[5] chronicled the events that nearly killed him. He was disappointed in the medical establishment's response to the changes in his life, changes that began with the moment of diagnosis. Some caring individuals attended him in the hospital, but Mullan turned to outside sources to restore his sense of self. Mullan's malignancy was "cured," but he continues to regard the life of cancer "survivors" as permanently affected by the illness.[6]

Although few have written extensively about it, other physi-

[4]J. Andrew Billings, *Outpatient Management of Advanced Cancer, Symptom Control, Support, and Hospice-in-the-Home* (Philadelphia: Lippincott, 1985).

[5]Fitzhugh Mullan, M.D., *Vital Signs* (New York: Farrar, Straus & Giroux, 1975).

[6]In league with Barbara Hoffman, Mullan has edited a book, *Charting the Journey*, that provides a sensitive, authoritative, balanced, and objective view of the experience of cancer from the time of diagnosis. It is well stocked with advice, addresses, and telephone numbers and should serve as a valuable guide to the perplexed. The National Coalition for Cancer Survivorship, the organization that produced *Charting the Journey* has taken on the serious task of helping cancer survivors reintegrate into society.

cians have shared the belief that personal narrative might help spread understanding of the experience of severe illness. Mandell and Spiro[7] asked fifty physicians to write narratives about their personal experiences with severe illnesses. *When Doctors Get Sick*, an edited collection of these narratives, covers a broad range of diseases. It includes stories by eleven physicians who had cancer, most of whom survived. The physician-authors viewed themselves as if they had been forced to cope in unfamiliar territory, as Mandell, in describing his own malignancy, relates

> Late one night when visitors had left, I talked at length with a patient in the room next to mine. At 27 she was dying of Hodgkin's disease and was well aware of her prognosis. Although I had passed the examinations put out by the American Board of Internal Medicine, she seemed to know a lot more about being sick than I did.[8]

Although written for physicians in sometimes technical terms, *When Doctors Get Sick* provides abundant evidence that, like patients in general, physician-patients encounter frustration, humiliation, diagnostic confusion, treatment failure, and unfeeling doctors and nurses. I found it useful reading because of the clarity with which the authors could identify the sources of their distress.

Progress in training physicians to listen and react to patients' concerns about their illnesses has been slow, but the field has not been totally neglected. Indeed, psycho-oncologists, such as Holland and Rowland,[9] have developed a formal framework for the evaluation and treatment of psychiatric disorders in the context of cancer. A thoughtful, academic approach to psychiatric needs

[7]Harvey Mandell and Howard Spiro, *When Doctors Get Sick* (New York: Plenum, 1987).

[8]Ibid., p. 291.

[9]J. C. Holland and J. Rowland, eds., *Psycho-oncology: The Psychological Care of the Patient with Cancer* (New York: Oxford University Press, 1989).

is appropriate when the coping structure shows signs of failing, but what about normal coping mechanisms? How can nonpsychiatrists avert "emotional breakdown" by taking preventive action?

A sensitive monograph on the subject of giving effective emotional support to people with cancer was written by a practicing oncologist, Ernest Rosenbaum,[10] almost two decades ago. He depicted his relationships with several patients by giving extensive details of the caring relationship he established with them. Rosenbaum's respect for the persons he was treating proved to be central to the process of caring for them. Indeed, Dr. Rosenbaum's effectiveness at showing respect extended to engaging his patients as teachers of other patients and physicians.

Rosenbaum was part of a growing group of practicing physicians who have sought to convey the experience of a doctor–patient relationship that extends beyond the diagnosis and treatment of disease. Included among them is Eric Cassell,[11] who explored the gap between technological health care, which is almost a cult form among some American physicians, and the nontechnical approach to the troubling problems of people with severe illness. Rather than impose diagnoses and treatments for objectively defined disorders, Cassell argued forcefully that in seeking to heal human ailments, physicians should allow themselves to listen to their patients' complaints, to respond to their patients' feelings, to be the healers their patients seek instead of rigidly defining themselves on their own terms.

To be that sort of physician, I had to be willing to learn from my patients. Like other practitioners who love the art of medicine, I found my patients to be willing teachers. Some novices presume

[10]Ernest H. Rosenbaum, *Living with Cancer* (St. Louis: Mosby, 1982) [New York: New American Library, Plume Books].

[11]Eric J. Cassell, *The Healer's Art: A New Approach to the Doctor–Patient Relationship* (Philadelphia and New York: Lippincott, 1976); Eric J. Cassell, *The Nature of Suffering and the Goals of Medicine* (New York: Oxford University Press, 1991).

that such teaching ends with the completion of formal training. Seasoned physicians continue to learn from their patients every day. But it is unusual for experienced doctors to report on lessons learned in their mature years as Yalom did in *Love's Executioner*[12]. A professor of psychiatry at Stanford, Yalom described the process by which he learned about diagnostic and therapeutic errors by "listening" to patients. In so doing, he defined a central issue of the learning experience. Our own preconceptions can be handicaps. We need to hear more and judge less.

"Listening" is much more than a passive activity. It includes a willingness to hear information in the context of an individual's own perspective. In *The Illness Narratives*, Arthur Kleinman[13] has provided the theoretical underpinnings in an extensive study of the process by which physicians can incorporate the experience of illness. I share his view that one's own experience of an illness is of only minor importance in the listening-understanding process. Rather, I believe good listening enables us to appreciate the significance which illness has for people vastly different from ourselves.

Many books about the experience of cancer have been written by nonphysicians. Survivors have told success stories, from Herbert Howe's personal triumph through physical exercise[14] to Arthur Frank's more reflective views on the deeper meaning of serious illness in the life of a mature individual.[15] Like Mullan, Howe's experience with malignancy led to rapid emotional maturity with a consequent sensitivity to the needs of others. Frank, whose prior academic training in sociology enabled him to make analytical

[12]Irvin D. Yalom, *Love's Executioner* (New York: Basic Books, 1989).

[13]Arthur Kleinman, *The Illness Narratives: Suffering, Healing, and the Human Condition* (New York: Basic Books, 1988).

[14]Herbert Howe, *Do Not Go Gentle* (New York: Norton, 1981).

[15]Arthur Frank, *At the Will of the Body* (Boston: Houghton Mifflin, 1991).

observations, described the complex effects of malignancy on his personal relationships. His emphasis on language was of particular interest to me.

Anatole Broyard[16] wrote essays relating to his experience with prostate cancer (his father's and his own). Broyard regarded the crisis of fatal illness as an artistic challenge. He used vivid prose to outlast his anticipated death.[17] As a literary critic for the *New York Times*, he had a reputation for originality, insight, and objectivity. *Intoxicated by My Illness* has all these qualities and includes reviews of several books written about death. In few words Broyard says much.

Optimists, such as Norman Cousins,[18] developed an enthusiastic following of nonphysicians eager to take responsibility for their sense of well-being. Carl Simonton, Stephanie Matthews-Simonton, and James L. Creighton,[19] Bernie Siegel,[20] and Lawrence LeShan[21] advocate the use of emotional interventions to help control cancer. The subject remains controversial because there is little scientific evidence to support it. The issue has recently been explored by Christopher Peterson and Lisa M. Bossio.[22]

I believe we oncologists are responsible for listening well to all of our patients, whether they are optimists or pessimists. We ought not to judge the quality of the effort our patients are making to

[16]Anatole Broyard, *Intoxicated by My Illness and Other Writings on Life and Death* (New York: Clarkson Potter, 1992).

[17]Broyard coped with fatal illness because he could retain his sense of self; he remained a writer and a critic. In contrast, Jack J. Lewis (one of the physician-patients in *When Doctors Get Sick*), although relatively dispassionate about his death from leukemia, was severely depressed about his inability to continue being a physician.

[18]Norman Cousins, *Anatomy of an Illness as Perceived by the Patient* (New York: Norton, 1979).

[19]O. Carl Simonton, Stephanie Matthews-Simonton, and James L. Creighton, *Getting Well Again* (Los Angeles: Tarcher, 1978).

[20]Bernie H. Siegel, *Love, Medicine, and Miracles* (New York: Harper & Row, 1986).

[21]Lawrence LeShan, Ph.D., *Cancer as a Turning Point* (New York: Dutton, 1989).

[22]Christopher Peterson and Lisa M. Bossio, *Health and Optimism: New Research on the Relationship Between Positive Thinking and Physical Well-Being* (New York: The Free Press, 1991).

"get well." Rather, it is our obligation to respond to their ailments and to discover the context within which they view their malignancies, their illnesses, and their lives.

The lessons I have learned about listening are not unique to oncologists, to cancer, or to the friends and relatives of people who have cancer. They apply broadly to humans in distress, to people who have been afflicted, to members of our community who have suffered losses.

The lessons I have learned are scarcely new. They are all in the Book of Job. Given the time to talk and an attentive audience, people in distress can be remarkably articulate.

ACKNOWLEDGMENTS

ALTHOUGH this book was written by a single author, it is in the truest sense a collaborative effort. Not only have I learned most of what I have written by listening to the concerns of people with cancer and their families and friends, but many of them have suggested ideas, relationships, lines, and phrases that they believed deserved special emphasis in this work.

Thus, to my patients, my *essential collaborators* in the creation of *A Time to Hear, A Time to Help*, I owe the deepest gratitude.

I also owe a debt to the many teachers who contributed to my formal education. Among the faculty at the University of Chicago, Dr. Stanley Yachnin, in whose laboratory I worked for four years, held me to the high standards and academic ideals of that great institution. My interest in hematology and oncology was further stimulated by Drs. Howard H. Hiatt, Stephen Robinson, and Stuart Schlossman at the Beth Israel Hospital in Boston, by the late Dr. Carl V. Moore, and by Drs. Elmer Brown, Philip W. Majerus, Stuart Kornfeld, Virginia Minnich, Edward Reinhart, and Stanford Wessler at Washington University in St. Louis. Since I entered practice, I have been the happy beneficiary of the community outreach program of the Johns Hopkins Oncology Center, under the leadership of Drs. Martin Abeloff, Raymond Lenhardt, and Philip Waalkes. Another member of the Hopkins faculty, Dr. Stuart Grossman, provided thought-provoking criticism of the initial draft of this book.

Two rabbis, Balfour Brickner and Eugene Lipman, were responsible for the lion's share of my formal religious training. Their insight into human needs has been more meaningful to me than words can say.

Dr. S. Ralph Himmelhoch, whose early death still leaves an emptiness in my life, served as my mentor in the laboratory at the National Cancer Institute. His scholarship and love of literature were potent forces in shaping my interest in the humane side of medicine.

Peter Porosky taught me the elements of creative writing and edited earlier versions of this work. His book *How to Find Your Own Voice** enhanced my understanding of the emotional impact of various styles of writing. Under Peter's direction, members of the Sligo Creek Writers' Group also critiqued my early efforts.

My professional colleagues have taught me much of what I know. I have been fortunate to work in a community with many caring physicians. My partners, Drs. Richard H. Pollen, Eugene P. Libre, Jeremy V. Cooke, and K. Siena Kirwin, deserve special mention. Dr. Pollen's comments on the manuscript were particularly apt. Jean Muir, a certified oncology nurse, whose kindness and professionalism justifiably won her the Lane Adams award from the American Cancer Society, coordinates the nursing services in our office and has, from our first encounter, been a persuasive force in my life. I could not have undertaken the challenge of writing a book while continuing in full-time practice without the able support of Sharon Bono, Sandra Pisciotta, and Sandra Whittaker, leaders of our office crew, together with Cathy Bodine, Judith Cardelli, Kelly Culp, Gail Kline, Carol McKenzie, Patricia Muir, Steve Richards, and Cathy Wells.

*Peter Porosky, *How to Find Your Own Voice* (Lanham, Md.: University Press of America, 1986).

An important dimension was added to *A Time to Hear, A Time to Help* through my work with the Comprehensive Cancer Program at Suburban Hospital in Bethesda, Maryland. I owe a special debt of gratitude to Sharon Metzger, Nancy Endler, Betsy August, Jody Nurik, and the oncology nurses on 5C. Deborah Skolnik, the hospital librarian, helped me obtain reference material.

Friends in my community, Carey Bourke Tenen and Joseph Goodwin, gave suggestions and encouragement. Herb and Norma Marder and other residents of Monhegan gave ear and returned useful criticism. Donald Holden nurtured me through the pangs of the late drafts and helped me laugh when I began to take my work too seriously.

A Time to Hear, A Time to Help would not have found its way to publication as easily or well without the specific assistance of Leon Kass, to whom I am most grateful. Carolyn Magionelli was invaluable in transcription of the manuscript.

In the course of publishing my work, I have been supported by many people who shared my interest in helping people with cancer. My literary agent, Charlotte Sheedy, gave me much valued advice. Holly Pemberton, assistant in the offices of The Free Press, read my drafts with a sensitive and caring eye. My editor, Erwin Glikes, guided me through revisions of my manuscript with the delicacy of a skilled surgeon.

Family and friends have given valued support. Bess Bauer, Karen Featherman, and Nettie Rosenblum nurtured my interest in writing, as did Marilyn Greenwald and Ted Brody. Donald and Ruth Levine, Ray and Helen Faye Rosenblum, and Sara Brody provided particular insight and encouragement in the formation of this work. Lynda Goldsmith made pertinent suggestions. Eleanor Johnson, Twig Johnson, Carol Shulman, Sara Mazie, and Shelly Samuels took a strong interest in my ideas and helped them to mature.

I owe much to my uncles, Marc Rosenblum and Lawrence Goldsmith, who have witnesed this work from its inception, provided useful ideas, and insisted on high standards.

Sabbath dinners at our house have often become mini literary groups. Minnon Friedman and Elizabeth Bass read my earliest efforts. My mother, Janeth Rosenblum, an avid and effective reader, influenced me beyond measure, always tempering her pride in my creative efforts with critical objectivity.

My children, Rachel, Hank, and Sarah, provided strength and optimism, sensitivity and intelligence, raucous humor and a healthy sense of skepticism about their father's ability to comprehend the "important" things in life.

My wife, Flo, deserves more than a few words added to the bottom of a long list. Not only is Flo an astute reader and editor, but she is always willing to take time to hear, to be gracious under fire, to be kind and generous, to live at siege, and to prepare for the next disaster in the wake of one just past. She lives to love and loves to help, characteristics that have attracted the attention of many. I count myself fortunate to have been among the favored.

Index

Persons Diagnosed

Subject Index